MAIN-COURSE
VEGETARIAN
PLEASURES

Also by Jeanne Lemlin

Quick Vegetarian Pleasures

Vegetarian Pleasures: A Menu Cookbook

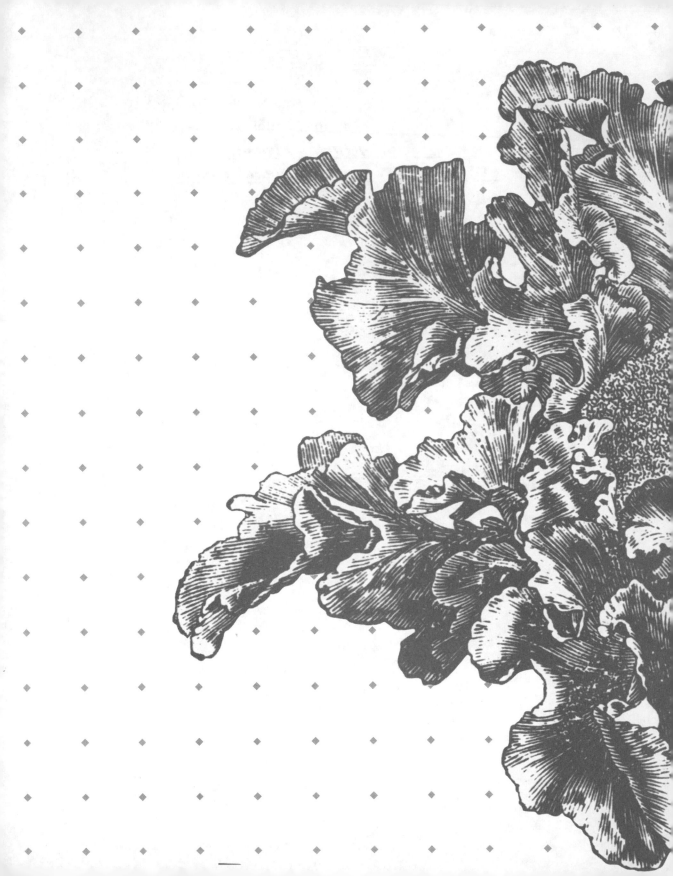

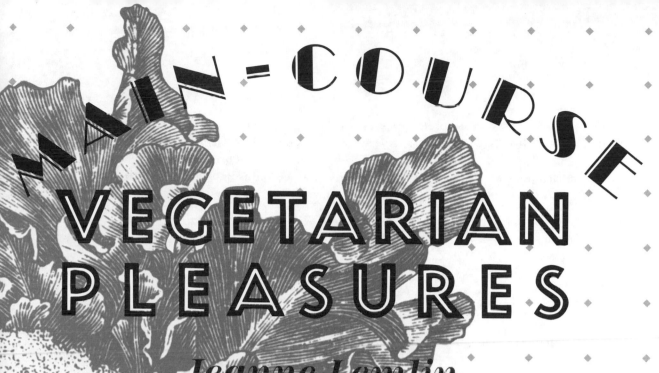

MAIN-COURSE
VEGETARIAN PLEASURES

Jeanne Lemlin

HarperPerennial
A Division of HarperCollins Publishers

HarperCollins books may be purchased for educational, business, or sales promotional use. For information please write: Special Markets Department, HarperCollins Publishers, Inc., 10 East 53rd Street, New York, NY 10022.

FIRST EDITION

Designed by Stephanie Tevonian

Library of Congress Cataloging-in-Publication Data

Lemlin, Jeanne.
    Main-course vegetarian pleasures / Jeanne Lemlin. — 1st ed.
      p.   cm.
    Includes index.
    ISBN 0-06-095022-6
  TX837.L447   1995
  641.5'636—dc20   94-23966

95 96 97 98 99 ❖/RRD 10 9 8 7 6 5 4 3 2 1

▼▼▼▼▼▼▼▼▼▼▼▼▼▼

To Susanne and Daniel,
two wonderful children who have given me so much joy

CONTENTS

ACKNOWLEDGMENTS

Many friends have given me suggestions and ideas that have been brought to play in the development of my recipes. Trips to restaurants recounted, new recipes discovered, dishes that they fantasized about, have all been food for my imagination. I would like to thank the following people who have contributed to this book, sometimes unbeknownst to them: Bonnie and Bob Benson for use of their "library," Stephanie Blumenthal, Billie Chernicoff, Julianne Lemlin, Rita Lemlin, Sally Patterson, Geri Rybacki, Mary Jane Simigan, David Tucker, Jane Walsh, and Christine Ward.

And a special thanks to my editor, Susan Friedland, for her continuous support.

INTRODUCTION

When it comes to preparing a vegetarian meal, the entrée is the biggest challenge. Favorite recipes for meatless appetizers, soups, salads, and, of course, breads and desserts are discovered in all types of cookbooks, as well as in magazines or from friends. But an exceptional vegetarian main course, that's a rarer bird. For many cooks, vegetarian and nonvegetarian alike, the meatless centerpiece that is outstanding and memorable is a real find.

So I have decided, in this third book of mine, to face the challenge head-on and offer you 125 recipes for vegetarian main courses. Most are quick and easy, and are so designated. Although my passion for cooking has not diminished over the years, I do have less time for it now with a young child to care for. Quickness, without sacrificing quality, has become the pace in my kitchen. My idea of a quick meal is preparation time of less than thirty minutes. I don't include baking or marinating time because nothing is demanded of me except waiting.

There are occasions, however, when I want to extend myself and prepare an elaborate meal for guests. I've included these more involved dishes in the Especially for Entertaining chapter. Although they demand more attention, they are generally not difficult to prepare. And in many instances you can prepare some of the steps in advance.

As in my second book, *Quick Vegetarian Pleasures*, I have maintained a cautious but relaxed approach to health and diet. Although I am watchful of my fat intake, and I cook with a plentiful assortment of fresh vegetables, grains, and legumes, I have avoided turning my recipes into mathematical problems by calculating all the nutrients and fats. I lament the trend in today's cooking where the kitchen no longer seems a place of joy, comfort, and fun but instead a laboratory in which food has become a problem to be solved. In so many kitchens, cans of vegetable-oil spray now take up counter space next to the calculator.

Sometimes it feels as though the "fat patrol" is out there ready to flagel-late those food writers who don't provide nutritional breakdowns with their recipes. Some writers have become so intimidated by this expectation that they artificially keep these figures down by increasing the number of portions a recipe will serve. Smaller portions mean lower fat figures. This is deceptive.

The servings in this book are generous. For example, a large pizza, a pound of pasta, a main-course grain or pasta salad usually will serve four people in my family. Most cookbooks, however, would say these dishes serve six. Six mouselike portions, perhaps, not genuinely satisfying ones.

The moderate approach to eating has always worked well for me. I choose lower-fat meals most of the time and allow myself to indulge in richer foods on occasion. Dessert is not an everyday treat; instead, I eat it only occasionally and make certain that it is worth waiting for. Brunch is another time when I allow myself to splurge. It is not a meal I often prepare, but when I do, richer foods seem to suit the occasion. Foods very low in fat just don't provide the comforting touch one expects from a brunch, and so in those rare instances I relax my guard. With this approach I never feel deprived of the pleasures of eating, and the kitchen doesn't become a battlefield. But each person has to decide what works best for him or her and carry out that plan.

Eating and cooking are highly personal matters. Tastes are like fingerprints—no two are exactly alike. But one's tastes can change with education and exposure to new foods. The best way to develop an appreciation for fresh, wholesome food is to cook with these ingredients using adventurous, well-tested recipes that put flavor above all else. Once you begin to prepare meatless meals with grains, vegetables, and/or beans taking center stage, then any mystery surrounding them dissolves, and they soon become familiar additions to your cooking repertory. Couscous, polenta, assorted beans and lentils, lots of fresh vegetables, and sundry pastas can become the building blocks for a new way of eating, providing seemingly endless variety and enjoyment.

If our diets are composed principally of generous amounts of fresh, healthful foods, then allowing ourselves a shortcut here and there does not compromise our standards in any significant measure. For example, frozen vegetables such as kale, spinach, peas, and corn can be great time-savers for the busy cook without sacrificing flavor or texture. Canned beans are another example. If I allowed myself only freshly cooked beans rather than canned versions when pressed for time, I would eat far fewer beans. Cooking beans from scratch takes time and forethought, and with my busy schedule I know I would, more often than not, seek other, quicker recipes if I had to begin a recipe by cooking beans. So this is an allowance I grant myself, and I eat a lot more beans as a result. I do recommend, however, that you snoop around and find brands that don't have a preservative in them. They do exist (at both supermarkets and natural foods stores), and you'll find they are just as good, if not better, than those with disodium EDTA added.

Above all, I want you to enjoy your time in the kitchen. My three books have kept the words "Vegetarian Pleasures" in their titles because the pleasurable aspect of cooking is what is most in danger of being lost with the waxing and waning of so many cooking trends. Preserving that pleasure is of central importance to me. Whether you are a vegetarian or are just tired of having meat as the center of each meal, these recipes are meant to awaken your palate to a new sense of vegetable-based cookery. So with an eye on good health and with pleasure as our guide, let's begin to cook.

A NOTE ON ORGANIZATION

Many of the recipes in this book would fit equally well in different chapters, and so I would like to explain why they are where they are. For example, Baked Vegetables with Garlic, White Beans, and Olives could be in the vegetable chapter as well as the bean chapter. I chose to place it in the bean chapter because the beans give the dish a special character and they come to mind first when I think of that dish. When recipes can be categorized a number of ways, I have generally relied on the strongest association the recipe conjures up to help define it. Because of the inevitable arbitrariness of some of the placements, it is a good idea to check the index as well as the individual chapters if you are looking for a specific recipe or want to cook with a certain ingredient.

NOTES ON INGREDIENTS

To make your meal planning easier, stock your cupboards with the following nonperishable items; you'll find that your work in the kitchen will be simplified immensely:

- couscous
- cornmeal
- white and brown rice
- bulghur
- lentils, both red and brown
- canned chickpeas
- canned black, kidney, and pinto beans
- canned whole tomatoes and crushed tomatoes
- tamari soy sauce
- assorted pastas
- olive oil
- a favorite tomato sauce

I included an extensive glossary of ingredients in my first book, *Vegetarian Pleasures: A Menu Cookbook,* and a number of sidebars on ingredients in my second book, *Quick Vegetarian Pleasures.* In order to help you with shopping, I am going to repeat some of that information here.

BEANS To cook dried beans, either soak them overnight in plenty of water or boil them for 2 minutes and let them soak 1 hour in that water. They will then be ready to cook. Drain them, add plenty of fresh water, and cook at a lively simmer until tender. Canned beans vary in quality—some are overcooked and too soft, especially kidney beans. Try different brands, and look for ones without disodium EDTA added. Always rinse canned beans in a strainer before using them.

CHILI PASTE WITH GARLIC A concentrated mixture of ground chilies and garlic used in Chinese cooking. A little goes a long way. It can be found in most supermarkets and specialty food stores, and lasts a long time in the refrigerator.

COUSCOUS This "grain" is created by mixing semolina (coarse flour made from hard durum wheat) and water to form tiny granules. There's nothing quicker to cook than couscous; you just pour boiling stock or water on it and let it sit for 5 minutes. Do try the various recipes in this book using couscous; it has a delicate texture and flavor.

LENTILS, RED These tiny orange seeds are popular in Indian cooking. They cook quickly, turning a rich tan color. Their delicious, buttery flavor is enhanced when they are combined with Indian spices. They can be purchased in natural foods stores, specialty food shops, and Indian grocery stores.

MISO A naturally fermented Japanese soybean and/or grain purée that is filled with friendly bacteria and digestion-aiding enzymes. It comes in various colors and strengths. I prefer barley miso, which is sweet, mild, and light in color. Always dilute miso with a little water before adding it to stocks; this will prevent clumping. Purchase unpasteurized miso; it is found in the refrigerated section of natural foods stores.

OLIVES Can be divided into four basic categories—ripe (black) or unripe (green), and oil-cured or brine-cured. Generally speaking, brine-cured olives are saltier with a more assertive flavor than oil-cured varieties. Greek kalamata olives are a well-known example of brine-cured olives. My favorite oil-cured olives from France are soaking in an herb-strewn olive oil when I purchase them. This keeps them plump and moist. Many oil-cured olives are packed in a drier state, resulting in wrinkled skins. When I purchase such olives, I cover them with olive oil, herbs, and a generous slice of orange peel and store them in the refrigerator. After I've eaten all the olives, I use this delicious marinade in cooking, such as in a tomato-garlic sauce for pasta or drizzled on French bread slices.

RED BELL PEPPERS I am including a note on these flaming wonders because they enhance so many dishes with their vibrant color and flavor. Red bell peppers are green peppers that have ripened on the bush. They are not at all spicy or hot. I have found a way to avoid their oftentimes outrageous price in the market, and I want to pass it on to you.

In August or September, when they are most abundant and at their lowest cost, I purchase large quantities and freeze them. They can be frozen raw, which preserves some of their crunchiness and saves a lot of time. Just core the peppers and remove the inner white membrane that is attached. Cut the peppers into large chunks, small dice, or thin strips. Place one cut-up pepper in a small freezer bag and push out as much air as possible before sealing. Freeze flat so that the pepper pieces are spread out and can freeze evenly. When you need one red pepper in a recipe, just remove one bag from the freezer. Let it thaw, then pat the pepper pieces dry before using them. They will have lost some of their crunchiness, so cook them less than you would fresh peppers.

SESAME OIL Oriental sesame oil is dark brown, strong-flavored, and made from toasted sesame seeds. It is not the same as light-colored, cold-pressed sesame oil found in natural foods stores. Oriental sesame oil has a hauntingly good flavor for which there is no substitute. It lasts indefinitely in the cupboard, so always keep some on hand. It can be purchased in most supermarkets, specialty food stores, natural foods stores, and Asian grocery stores.

SOBA These long, flat Japanese noodles made from buckwheat cook quickly and are rather delicate, so take care not to overcook them. Their nutty flavor is unique and might take a little getting used to. Although soba is expensive, I think it is well worth the price.

TAMARI SOY SAUCE Tamari (and shoyu soy sauce made from soy and wheat) is an aged soy sauce that has a full-bodied flavor and is preservative-free. It can be purchased in natural foods stores and will last indefinitely in the refrigerator.

TEMPEH Ground soybeans and a living culture are fermented and then pressed into a cake to form tempeh. Like most soybean products, it is packed with nutrients: protein, iron, and vitamin B-12. When it is fresh, there are oftentimes black spots on it. These are part of the tempeh and are harmless. When tempeh is spoiled it will have an acrid smell, be slimy, and have blue, green, pink, or yellow mold on it. Tempeh must be cooked before eating. Because it freezes so well, it is easy to always have some on hand. Tempeh can be purchased in natural foods stores.

TOFU Also called bean curd, tofu is a type of soybean cheese. Soybeans are cooked and mashed, then their liquid (soy milk) is pressed out of them and mixed with a coagulant to separate the curds from the whey. The curds are then pressed into cakes to form tofu. It is an excellent source of protein and iron, and a good source of calcium. I always purchase extra-firm tofu because I prefer its texture. To fry tofu, you must pat the pieces very dry with paper or cotton towels, or else the tofu will stick to the pan. If you are using a cast-iron pan and you heat the oil until it is very hot (but not smoking), it is unlikely the tofu will stick. Using a nonstick pan is also an easy way to get crisp, perfectly fried tofu.

TORTILLAS These thin Mexican "pancakes" vary greatly from brand to brand. Some brands make thick, dry tortillas that break easily; others produce flaky, delicate ones. Flour tortillas, especially, need to be moist and supple. Try different brands, and when you discover a winner, freeze a few packages so you will have them on hand.

VEGETABLE STOCK

I rarely make my own vegetable stock because of the time and forethought needed to prepare a full-bodied stock. I purchase powdered vegetable stock base from my local health food store, and it makes a delicious stock. Most supermarket brands have ingredients in their stocks that you can't pronounce—beware! Powdered stock base or cubes last a long time in the refrigerator, so you can always have it available. Should you want to make your stock from scratch, here is a recipe for a delicious vegetable stock:

8 cups water

¼ cup tamari soy sauce

3 unpeeled carrots, washed and diced

3 celery ribs, diced

4 cups chopped cabbage

½ bunch parsley (stems included), chopped

3 onions, diced

6 garlic cloves, coarsely chopped

2 bay leaves

1 clove

Generous seasoning of freshly ground pepper

Dash of nutmeg

Makes 7 cups

1 Place everything in a large stockpot and bring to a boil. Reduce to a simmer and cook 1 hour, stirring occasionally.

2 Remove the bay leaves and discard. Strain the stock and discard the vegetables. Let the stock cool. Store in a tightly covered jar in the refrigerator, or pour into ice cube trays and freeze. When frozen, remove the cubes from the tray and store them in a plastic bag. Use as needed. The stock will stay fresh in the refrigerator for 1 week. After a week, bring the stock to a boil, then simmer for 10 minutes. The stock will keep fresh for 1 more week.

HEARTY SOUPS AND THICK STEWS

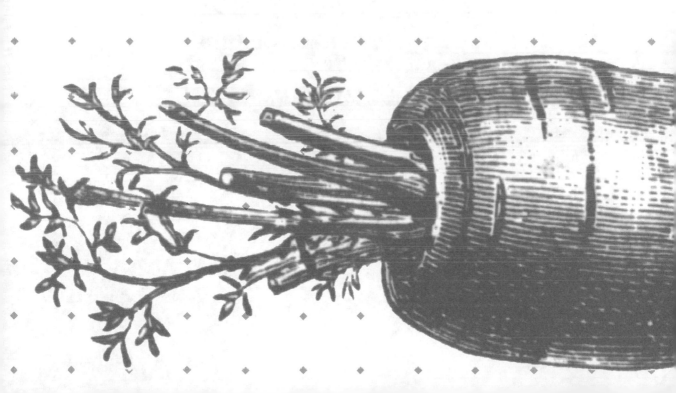

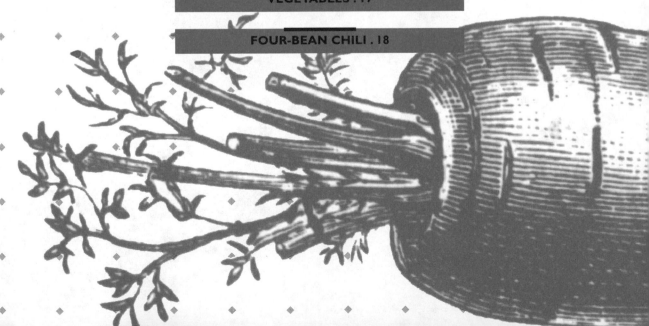

f you can spare an hour or so on weekends to make soup, you will benefit the whole week long. Soup improves as it stands, and most of these recipes produce a large pot, which enables you to freeze a portion. Soup lasts a number of days in the refrigerator and it reheats well, making it possible for you to get a few meals out of one batch. For convenience, soup can't be beat.

To make a great soup, you have to follow a few rules. When onions and garlic are called for, they must be sautéed before any liquid is added. This heightens their flavors and gives the soup dimension. If you were to just drop the onions and garlic into the stock, you'd have a weak-flavored soup. Also, make an effort to find a good vegetable stock base, whether powdered or

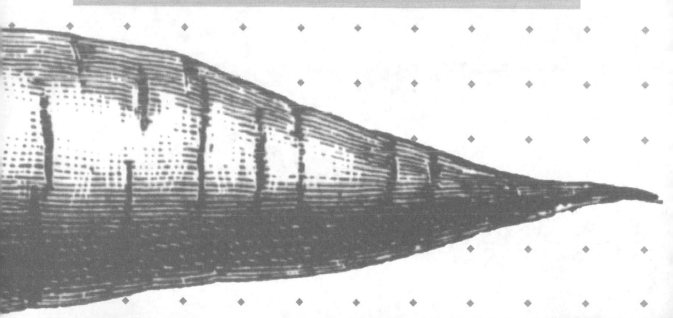

cubed, or make your own stock, for stock is the foundation from which all the other flavors build.

I try to prepare my soups at least a few hours in advance, but preferably the day before. Freshly made soup often lacks depth, and just a few hours of sitting can make it swim with flavor.

These soups are substantial and are meant to be main courses. If you serve a tantalizing salad made with assorted greens and some whole grain or crusty French bread alongside, you'll have a heavenly, wholesome meal.

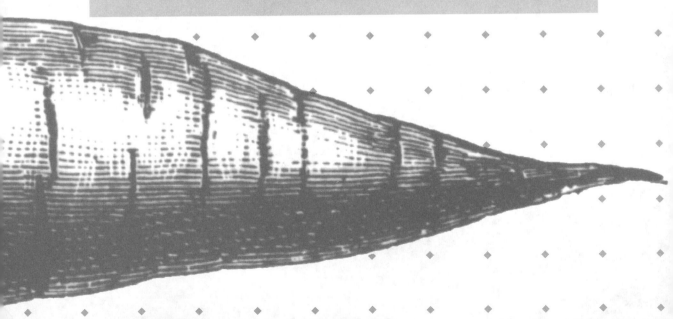

PUMPKIN AND CORN CHOWDER

Cooked pumpkin, a great source of beta carotene, is very mild and it gives wonderful body and color to this delicious chowder. Don't hesitate to make this soup a few days in advance because, as with most soups, it benefits from sitting.

2 medium-large leeks

¼ cup olive oil

2 carrots, finely diced

10 cups vegetable stock

2 medium boiling potatoes, peeled and finely diced

1 ½ teaspoons salt

Generous seasoning of freshly ground pepper

¼ teaspoon ground cloves

Dash of cayenne

2 16-ounce cans pumpkin

½ cup heavy cream

2 cups fresh or frozen corn kernels

Minced fresh parsley for garnish

Serves 6 as a main course

1 Cut the root ends off the leeks. Cut a slit vertically along the entire length of each leek, cutting *almost* all the way through to the back. Rinse the leeks under cold running water, flipping through each layer to look for any hidden dirt. Thinly slice the white part of each leek plus about 3 inches of the green part. You should have about 3 cups.

2 Heat the olive oil in a large stockpot over medium heat. Add the leeks and carrots and sauté for 15 minutes. Pour in the vegetable stock and bring to a boil. Add the potatoes, salt, pepper, cloves, and cayenne; cook the soup for 30 minutes.

3 Place the pumpkin in a large bowl. Ladle about a cup of soup onto the pumpkin and stir it together to liquefy it. Pour it into the soup along with the heavy cream and corn. Cook 5 more minutes (or longer if the chowder is too thin). Serve in bowls with minced parsley sprinkled on top.

ROASTED RED PEPPER SOUP WITH DILL DUMPLINGS

§tart this tasty soup early in the day so all you'll have to do at dinnertime is drop in the dumplings. And when you purée the soup, use a blender, if possible, rather than a food processor for a silkier finish.

4 to 5 large (2 pounds) red bell peppers (or 2 cups purchased roasted red peppers)

3 tablespoons olive oil

4 garlic cloves, minced

2 onions, finely diced

6 cups vegetable stock, plus more for thinning soup

1 celery rib, thinly sliced

2 carrots, thinly sliced

2 medium potatoes, peeled and finely diced

1 teaspoon salt

Generous seasoning of freshly ground pepper

Dash of cayenne

1½ tablespoons balsamic or red wine vinegar

DILL DUMPLINGS

1 cup unbleached flour

1¾ teaspoons baking powder

½ teaspoon salt

1 teaspoon sugar

1 Roast the peppers on a baking sheet close to the flame or heating element of a broiler. As they blacken, turn with tongs until evenly charred all over. This will take about 20 minutes. When done, place the peppers in a plastic bag and close the bag. Let them steam 10 minutes. Remove and discard the cores and seeds of the peppers, then peel off the blackened skin. (This can be done under cold running water.) Pat the peppers dry with paper towels. Dice the peppers; you should get at least 2 cups. If you are using purchased roasted peppers, dice them.

2 Heat the olive oil in a large stockpot. Add the garlic and onions and cook until the onions begin to brown, about 15 minutes.

3 Add the stock, celery, carrots, potatoes, salt, pepper, and cayenne. Bring the soup to a boil, then reduce to a simmer. Cook for about 20 minutes, or until the vegetables are tender. Stir in the reserved roasted peppers and cook 10 more minutes.

4 Let the soup cool 10 minutes, then purée it in batches in a blender or food processor. Return it all to the large pot. (The soup must be in a large, wide pot so there's room to cook the dumplings.) Stir in the vinegar, then stir in enough stock to

1½ teaspoons minced fresh dill, or 1 teaspoon dried

1 tablespoon chilled butter

¾ cup cold low-fat milk

....

2 tablespoons minced fresh parsley

Serves 4 to 6 as a main course

thin the soup to a heavy-cream consistency. The soup will thicken while the dumplings cook in it.

5 To make the dumplings, combine the flour, baking powder, salt, sugar, and dill in a medium-size bowl. Cut the butter into bits, then toss it into the flour mixture. With your fingertips, rub the butter into the flour until it forms coarse crumbs. Stir in the milk just until blended. Cover and chill the dumpling batter for 30 minutes, or up to 1½ hours.

6 Return the soup to a boil. Reduce the heat to a simmer. Drop in teaspoonfuls of dumpling batter to form 1½-inch dumplings (you should have about 16). Immediately cover the pot and simmer the soup 10 minutes, or until the dumplings are puffed. Do not remove the cover until the 10 minutes are up. Serve the soup with some dumplings in each bowl and garnish with parsley.

VEGETABLE CHOWDER

You can't beat the flavor or the great palette of colors in this chowder.

2 tablespoons unsalted butter

2 onions, very finely diced

3 garlic cloves, minced

½ pound mushrooms, thinly sliced (3 cups)

5 cups vegetable stock

2 carrots, thinly sliced

2 celery ribs, thinly sliced

2 cups finely shredded cabbage

1 medium-size potato, peeled and thinly sliced into bite-size pieces

2 tablespoons converted white rice

1 medium-size zucchini, quartered lengthwise and thinly sliced

½ cup fresh or frozen corn kernels

2 tablespoons minced fresh basil, or 1½ teaspoons dried

3 cups milk

½ cup heavy cream

½ teaspoon salt

Liberal seasoning of freshly ground pepper

Serves 4 as a main course

1 Heat the butter in a large stockpot over medium heat. Add the onions and garlic and sauté for 5 minutes. Stir in the mushrooms and sauté 10 minutes more, stirring often.

2 Pour in the stock, then add the carrots, celery, cabbage, potato, and rice. Cook at a lively simmer for 20 minutes.

3 Add the zucchini, corn, and basil; cook for 10 minutes. Mix in the milk, cream, salt, and pepper and cook an additional 5 minutes, but don't let the soup boil. Remove 2 cups of soup and purée it in a blender or food processor. Return it to the pot. Taste for salt before serving.

BLACK BEAN SOUP

A *full-flavored, delicious soup that is smooth with bits of bean throughout. A salad with orange sections, black olives, and red onions would be a great starter.*

1 pound (about 2¼ cups) dried black beans

½ cup olive oil

4 garlic cloves, minced

3 medium-large onions, diced

2 teaspoons ground cumin

1 teaspoon dried oregano

2 bay leaves

1 green pepper, cored and diced

2 celery ribs, diced

¼ cup tomato sauce

½ cup chopped fresh parsley

10 cups vegetable stock

1 tablespoon apple cider vinegar

½ teaspoon Tabasco sauce

1½ teaspoons salt

Generous seasoning of freshly ground pepper

1 tablespoon cream sherry or sweet vermouth

Sour cream for garnish

Serves 4 as a main course

1 Rinse the beans in a colander, then place them in a large pot and cover with water. Let soak overnight. (Alternatively, bring the beans to a boil and cook for 2 minutes. Remove from the heat, cover the pot, and let soak 1 hour.) Drain the beans in a colander and set aside.

2 Heat the olive oil in a large stockpot over medium heat. Add the garlic, onions, cumin, oregano, and bay leaves and sauté for 10 minutes, stirring often.

3 Stir in the beans, green pepper, celery, tomato sauce, parsley, vegetable stock, vinegar, Tabasco, salt, and pepper. Bring to a boil, then reduce the heat to a lively simmer. Cook, uncovered, stirring occasionally, for 1½ hours, or until the beans are very tender. Discard the bay leaves.

4 Remove about 4 cups of the soup and purée it in a blender or food processor. Return it to the pot. Stir in the sherry and cook 5 minutes more. The soup should have a consistency similar to heavy cream; boil a few more minutes if it is too thin, add a little stock if too thick. Serve in bowls with a small dollop of sour cream on top; it doesn't need much.

Quick SWEET POTATO AND VEGETABLE STEW WITH FRESH GREENS

Sweet potatoes as the base of this stew not only lend a distinctive brilliance but also give it a wondrously rich flavor. If you are not fond of cilantro, just omit it, or substitute fresh parsley.

¼ cup olive oil

3 onions, finely diced

4 garlic cloves, minced

2 celery ribs, thinly sliced

8 cups vegetable stock or water

1½ cups finely chopped canned tomatoes with their juice

2 medium-large sweet potatoes, peeled and cut into 1-inch dice

1 carrot, thinly sliced

¼ teaspoon nutmeg

2 tablespoons minced cilantro (optional)

1½ teaspoons salt

Dash of cayenne

Generous seasoning of freshly ground pepper

5 cups (5 ounces) lightly packed fresh spinach, kale, or Swiss chard, torn into small pieces

Serves 4 to 6 as a main course

1 Heat the olive oil in a large stockpot over medium heat. Add the onions, garlic, and celery and sauté, stirring often, for 10 minutes. Stir in all of the remaining ingredients except the greens.

2 Bring the soup to a boil, then reduce the heat to a simmer. Cook, stirring occasionally, for 45 minutes, or until the sweet potatoes are tender. Remove 2 cups of the soup and purée it; then return it to the pot.

3 Stir in the spinach, kale, or Swiss chard and cook the soup about 5 more minutes, or until the greens are tender.

AUTUMN VEGETABLE SOUP

Root vegetables, winter squash, and kale combine to make a soup that evokes the essence of autumn and winter. If time allows, make it the day before; sitting will intensify these heartwarming flavors. As with most soups, this one cries out for peasant-style bread to serve alongside.

¼ cup olive oil

2 medium onions, finely diced

4 garlic cloves, minced

2 large parsnips, thinly sliced

2 carrots, thinly sliced

1 tiny (1 pound) butternut squash, peeled and cut into ½-inch dice (2 cups)

12 cups vegetable stock

2 medium red-skinned potatoes, cut into ½-inch dice

½ teaspoon dried thyme

1 teaspoon salt

Generous seasoning of freshly ground pepper

½ pound fresh kale (weight with stems), torn into tiny pieces (about 4 cups)

1 16-ounce can Great Northern (small white) beans, drained and rinsed

Serves 8 as a main course

1 Combine the oil, onions, and garlic in a large stockpot. Cook over medium-high heat for 5 minutes, stirring often.

2 Stir in the parsnips, carrots, and squash and sauté, stirring often, until the vegetables begin to brown, about 15 minutes. This step adds depth to the soup's flavor, so be certain not to skip it.

3 Stir in the stock, potatoes, thyme, salt, and pepper and bring the soup to a boil. Reduce to a simmer and cook about 45 minutes, or until the vegetables are tender.

4 Stir in the kale and beans and cook about 10 more minutes, or until the kale is tender. Remove about 3 cups of the soup and purée it in a blender or food processor. Return to the pot and stir to blend.

Quick CURRIED CAULIFLOWER AND POTATO SOUP

Here's a low-fat soup that's teeming with flavor. A spoonful of yogurt on top is indispensable, adding a delightful tang and welcome creaminess. Be careful with the cayenne: a little goes a long way.

1 tablespoon unsalted butter

1 tablespoon oil

2 garlic cloves, minced

2 medium onions, finely diced

1 red bell pepper, finely diced

2 celery ribs, thinly sliced

1 tablespoon curry powder

2 teaspoons ground coriander

1 teaspoon ground cumin

1 teaspoon turmeric

A few dashes of cayenne

1 medium-size (2 pounds) cauliflower, cut into small pieces

3 medium-size potatoes, peeled and finely diced

6 cups vegetable stock

1½ teaspoons salt

2 tablespoons minced cilantro (optional)

Plain yogurt (essential)

Serves 6 as a main course

1 Heat the butter and oil in a large stockpot over medium heat. Add the garlic and onions and sauté, tossing often, until the onions are tender and golden, about 10 minutes. Add the red pepper and celery and sauté 5 minutes.

2 Sprinkle on all the spices and stir to evenly coat the vegetables. Cook, stirring often, for 2 minutes to toast the spices. Stir in the cauliflower and potatoes and coat them well with the spices.

3 Pour in the stock and salt and raise the heat to high. Bring the soup to a boil, then reduce the heat to a simmer. Cook 20 minutes, or until the vegetables are tender.

4 Ladle half of the soup into a bowl or saucepan, purée it in a blender or food processor, then return it to the soup pot. Stir in the optional cilantro. Serve in bowls with a generous dollop of yogurt on top.

Quick LENTIL SOUP WITH SWEET POTATOES

ach one of my cook-books has a recipe for a different rendition of lentil soup, and I'd be hard-pressed to choose my favorite among them. In this tasty version, sweet potatoes lend a rich flavor as well as color, and their high vitamin A content gives this already nutritious soup an added boost.

¼ cup olive oil

4 garlic cloves, minced

2 large onions, diced

1 teaspoon dried thyme

2 bay leaves

10 cups vegetable stock

1¼ cups lentils

2 celery ribs, sliced

½ cup minced fresh parsley

¾ teaspoon salt

Liberal seasoning of freshly ground pepper

2 medium (1 pound) sweet potatoes, peeled and cut into ¾-inch dice

Serves 4 to 6 as a main course

1 Heat the oil in a large stockpot over medium heat. Add the garlic, onions, thyme, and bay leaves and sauté for 10 minutes.

2 Raise the heat to high. Stir in the stock, lentils, celery, ¼ cup of the parsley, salt, and pepper. Bring to a boil, then reduce the heat to a lively simmer. Cook, uncovered, for 30 minutes.

3 Add the sweet potatoes and cook 20 more minutes, or until the sweet potatoes are tender. Discard the bay leaves. Remove 2 cups of the soup and purée in a blender or food processor. Return it to the pot with the remaining ¼ cup parsley. Cook 1 more minute before serving.

MINESTRONE SOUP

This is the perfect soup to choose when you want something full-bodied yet low in fat. This recipe makes a big potful, so don't hesitate to cool off a portion thoroughly and freeze it for future use; you'll be glad you did.

¼ cup fruity olive oil

2 large onions, finely diced

6 garlic cloves, minced

1 28-ounce can tomatoes, finely chopped with their juice

12 cups (3 quarts) vegetable stock

1 carrot, thinly sliced

2 celery ribs, thinly sliced

1 cup diced green beans

1 medium potato, cut into ½-inch cubes

1 16-ounce can chickpeas, rinsed and drained

2 bay leaves

3 tablespoons chopped fresh basil, or 1½ teaspoons dried

1 teaspoon dried oregano

A few pinches of saffron

Generous seasoning of freshly ground pepper

1½ tablespoons tamari soy sauce

1 Heat the oil in a large stockpot over medium heat. Add the onions and garlic and sauté, stirring often, until tender, about 10 minutes.

2 Stir in the tomatoes and their juice and cook 5 minutes. Add all the remaining ingredients except the zucchini, pasta, and cheese, and bring to a boil. Reduce to a lively simmer and cook 30 minutes, stirring occasionally.

3 Add the zucchini and pasta and cook 5 to 10 more minutes, or until the pasta is just tender. Pass the Parmesan cheese at the table, if desired.

1 small to medium
zucchini, quartered
lengthwise and thinly
sliced

⅓ cup macaroni or
spaghetti broken into
1-inch pieces

Grated Parmesan cheese
(optional)

Serves 10 as a main course

Quick SOBA SOUP WITH VEGETABLES AND TOFU

Soba served in broth is a traditional Japanese dish. It is a great choice when you want something light and revitalizing.

8 ounces soba (buckwheat noodles; see note)

5 cups water

⅓ cup tamari soy sauce

2 carrots, very thinly sliced

½ pound firm tofu, cut into ½-inch cubes

½ cup miso (see note)

2 tablespoons Oriental sesame oil

2 scallions, very thinly sliced

Serves 3 to 4 as a main course

1 Bring 3 quarts of water to a boil and cook the soba about 5 minutes, or until al dente. Do not overcook it. Drain in a colander, rinse under cold running water, drain again, and set aside.

2 In the same pot, bring the 5 cups of water and the tamari to a boil. Drop in the carrots and simmer 5 minutes. Stir in the tofu and cook 1 minute. Place the miso in a bowl, then remove about ½ cup of the broth and stir it into the miso to dilute it. Pour the mixture into the broth. Remove the pot from the heat so the miso doesn't boil. Stir in the sesame oil.

3 Place some soba in large soup bowls and ladle the soup over it. Sprinkle on the scallions.

Note: Soba and miso can be purchased at natural foods stores. My favorite variety of miso is the light-colored sweet miso.

Quick CURRIED RED LENTIL SOUP WITH VEGETABLES

Prepare this soup at least 2 hours before serving so the flavors mingle to produce a rich-flavored soup. If you are not familiar with red lentils (they are actually tiny orange lentils), you'll be glad to discover this tasty legume. Red lentils cook quickly, turn a golden color, and have a wonderful buttery flavor.

6 cups water

1½ cups red lentils, rinsed

1 tablespoon vegetable oil

½ teaspoon salt

1 medium potato, peeled and cut into ½-inch dice

2 tablespoons butter

2 garlic cloves, minced

1 small red bell pepper, finely diced

1 celery rib, thinly sliced

1 apple, peeled, cored, and cut into ½-inch dice

1½ tablespoons curry powder

½ teaspoon ground cumin

Dash of cayenne

1 tablespoon tamari soy sauce

4 ounces fresh spinach, torn into tiny pieces (4 cups)

Serves 4 to 6 as a main course

1 Bring the water to a boil in a 3-quart saucepan. Stir in the lentils, oil, and salt. When the water returns to a boil, reduce the heat to a simmer. Cook 20 minutes, stirring often. Scrape off and discard any foam that accumulates.

2 Stir in the potato and cook 20 more minutes, stirring frequently.

3 Meanwhile, melt 1 tablespoon of the butter in a medium-size skillet over medium heat. Add the garlic and cook 2 minutes. Stir in the red pepper, celery, and apple and sauté until tender, about 10 minutes. Sprinkle on the curry powder, cumin, and cayenne and cook 2 minutes, stirring often.

4 Scrape the vegetable mixture into the soup. Add the tamari, spinach, and remaining tablespoon of butter. Cook about 10 more minutes, or until the soup is the consistency of heavy cream—not watery or pasty. Stir often. Let the soup sit a few hours before serving. Reheat and check the consistency. Add a bit more water if it is too thick.

Quick FOUR-BEAN CHILI

Here is a tempting variation on chili that has vegetables in it. As with traditional chili, corn bread is the perfect accompaniment. Don't hesitate to make this large portion if you are feeding only a few people. Leftover chili can be served as another meal a few days later, and a portion can also be frozen.

3 tablespoons oil

2 large onions, diced

4 garlic cloves, minced

1 tablespoon chili powder

1 tablespoon ground cumin

½ teaspoon dried oregano

⅛ teaspoon cayenne

1 28-ounce can imported plum tomatoes, finely chopped with their juice

1 6-ounce can tomato paste

6 cups water

1 tablespoon tamari soy sauce

½ teaspoon salt

Freshly ground pepper

2 carrots, thinly sliced

2 green peppers, cored and diced

1 15-ounce can kidney beans, rinsed and drained

1 15-ounce can pinto beans, rinsed and drained

1 15-ounce can chickpeas, rinsed and drained

1 Heat the oil in a large stockpot over medium heat. Add the onions and garlic and sauté 10 minutes. Sprinkle in the chili powder, cumin, oregano, and cayenne. Cook, stirring constantly, for 2 minutes.

2 Stir in the tomatoes, tomato paste, water, tamari, salt, and pepper and blend well. Bring to a boil over medium-high heat, then add the carrots and green peppers. Cook, stirring occasionally, until the carrots are tender, about 30 minutes.

3 Add the beans and zucchini and cook until the zucchini is tender, about 10 more minutes. If the chili is too thin, cook a little longer; if it is too thick, add a bit more water. Stir in the butter just before serving.

1 15-ounce can black beans, rinsed and drained

1 medium zucchini, diced

1 tablespoon unsalted butter

Serves 6 to 8 as a main course

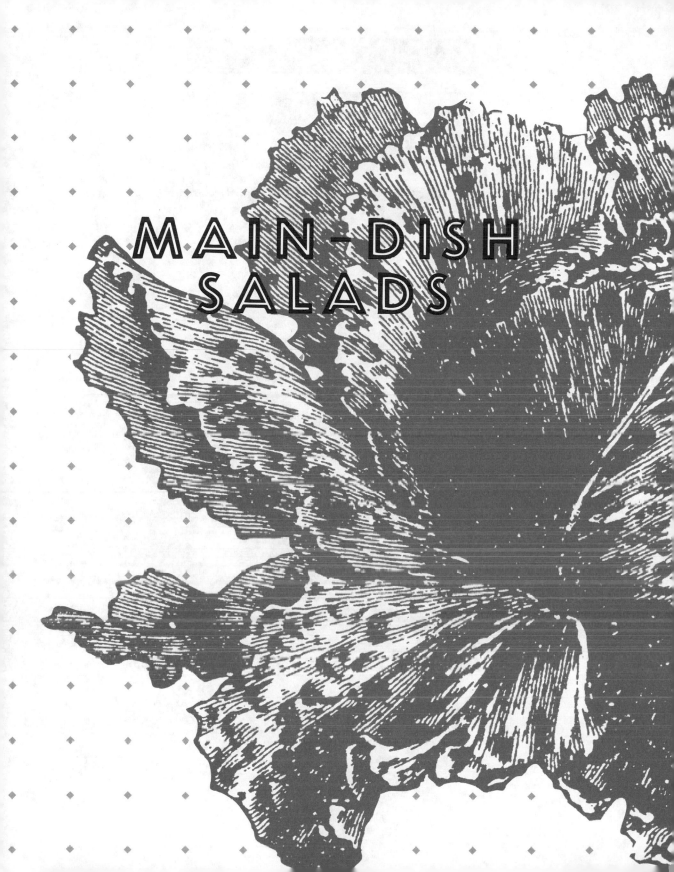

MAIN-DISH SALADS

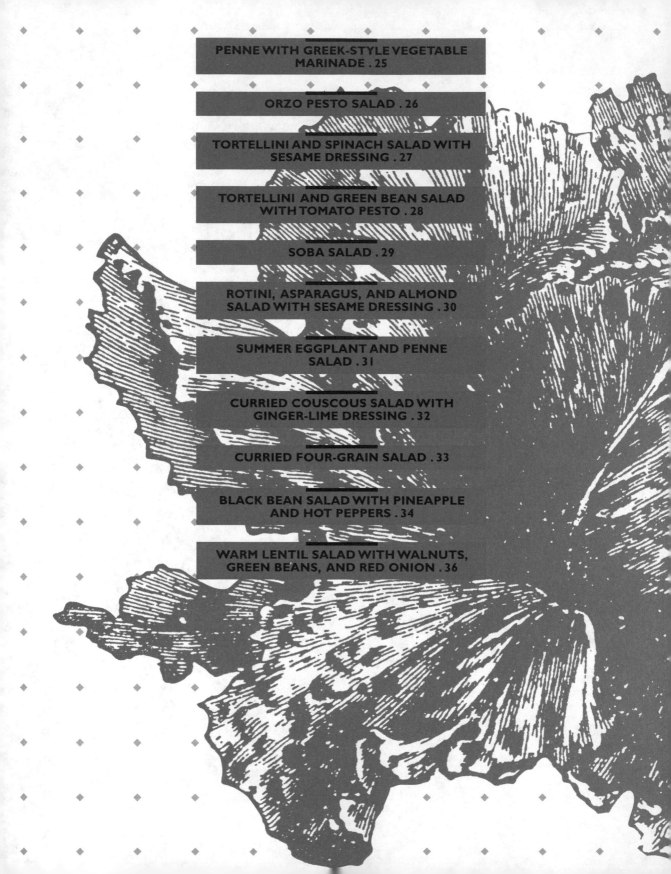

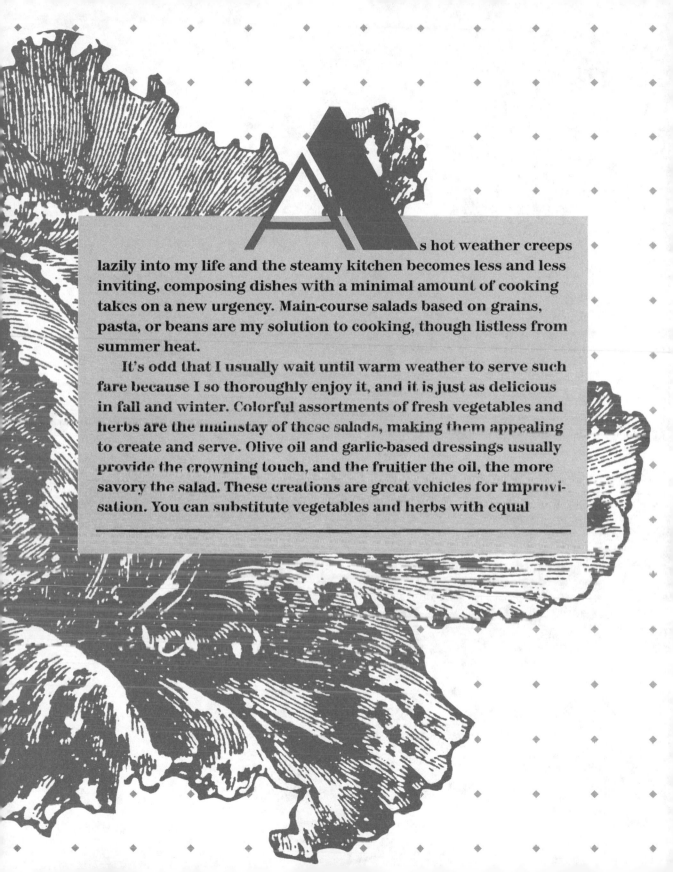

As hot weather creeps lazily into my life and the steamy kitchen becomes less and less inviting, composing dishes with a minimal amount of cooking takes on a new urgency. Main-course salads based on grains, pasta, or beans are my solution to cooking, though listless from summer heat.

It's odd that I usually wait until warm weather to serve such fare because I so thoroughly enjoy it, and it is just as delicious in fall and winter. Colorful assortments of fresh vegetables and herbs are the mainstay of these salads, making them appealing to create and serve. Olive oil and garlic-based dressings usually provide the crowning touch, and the fruitier the oil, the more savory the salad. These creations are great vehicles for improvisation. You can substitute vegetables and herbs with equal

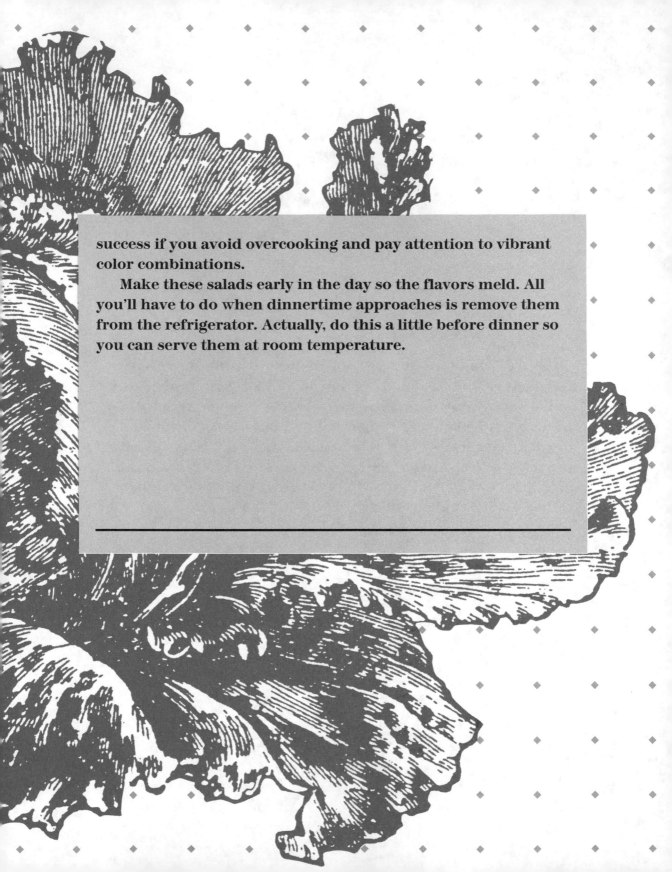

success if you avoid overcooking and pay attention to vibrant color combinations.

Make these salads early in the day so the flavors meld. All you'll have to do when dinnertime approaches is remove them from the refrigerator. Actually, do this a little before dinner so you can serve them at room temperature.

PENNE WITH GREEK-STYLE VEGETABLE MARINADE

Quick

This "sauce" requires no cooking; just marinate everything in one bowl and toss it onto the hot pasta. Great for summer because of the minimal amount of cooking involved.

⅓ cup olive oil

3 garlic cloves, pressed or minced

1 medium zucchini, halved lengthwise and very thinly sliced

2 tomatoes, finely diced

12 kalamata (Greek) olives, pitted and chopped (see note)

6 scallions, very thinly sliced

2 tablespoons finely chopped fresh dill, or 1½ teaspoons dried

1 cup finely diced feta cheese

Generous seasoning of freshly ground black pepper

1 pound penne or mostaccioli (quill-shaped pasta)

Salt to taste

Serves 6

1 Combine all the ingredients except the pasta and the salt in a medium-size bowl. Toss and let sit for 30 minutes or up to 4 hours. Cover and chill if held longer than 1 hour; bring to room temperature before cooking the pasta.

2 Bring a large pot of water to a boil. Add the pasta and cook until tender yet chewy, about 10 minutes. Drain thoroughly in a colander. Return to the pot or place in a large bowl.

3 Pour on the vegetable marinade and toss. Serve slightly warm or at room temperature, tasting to see if salt is necessary.

Note: To pit the olives, place them one by one on a cutting board. Lay the flat surface of a large chef's knife on the olive and give a thump with your fist. The pit will pop out. Cut the flesh into quarters.

Quick ORZO PESTO SALAD

Orzo salads pair particularly well with creamy dressings and this pesto sauce lends just the right balance, while diced vegetables and walnuts add some welcome crunch.

PESTO

1 well-packed cup fresh basil

¼ cup olive oil

3 garlic cloves, minced

½ teaspoon salt

Generous seasoning of freshly ground pepper

¼ cup grated Parmesan cheese

....

1½ cups orzo (rice-shaped pasta)

1 celery rib, thinly sliced

1 red bell pepper, finely diced

1 cucumber, peeled, seeded, and finely diced

⅓ cup slivered red onion

½ cup chopped walnuts

Serves 4

1 To make the pesto, combine the basil, olive oil, garlic, salt, and pepper in a blender or food processor and purée. Scrape into a bowl; stir in the Parmesan cheese. Set aside.

2 Cook the orzo in rapidly boiling water for 6 to 8 minutes, or until tender but not soft or mushy. Drain thoroughly in a colander, then place in a large bowl. Spoon on the pesto and toss well. Let cool.

3 Stir in the remaining ingredients, breaking up any clumps of orzo. Cover and chill at least 2 hours. Bring to room temperature before serving.

TORTELLINI AND SPINACH SALAD WITH SESAME DRESSING

Fresh spinach adds
*wonderful color and texture to this special
salad. Sesame lovers take note.*

SESAME DRESSING

⅓ cup canola oil

2 tablespoons Oriental sesame oil

2 tablespoons lemon juice

1 teaspoon tamari soy sauce

2 garlic cloves, minced

½ teaspoon salt

Freshly ground pepper

·····································

1 pound frozen cheese tortellini

1 yellow bell pepper, cut into thin strips

1 tomato, cut into small cubes

⅓ cup slivered red onion

2 teaspoons sesame seeds

4 cups fresh spinach torn into small pieces, washed and spun dry

Serves 4

1 Combine all the ingredients for the sesame dressing in a screw-top jar and shake vigorously. Set aside.

2 Bring a large pot of water to a boil. Drop in the tortellini and cook until al dente, about 5 minutes. Do not overcook. Drain in a colander. Run cold water over the tortellini until they are cold, then drain again very well. Pour into a large serving bowl.

3 Stir in the pepper, tomato, and onion, then pour on half of the sesame dressing and toss well. Let marinate at least 30 minutes, or up to 8 hours. Cover and chill if longer than 1 hour. Bring to room temperature before serving.

4 Place the sesame seeds in a dry, small saucepan and toast them over medium heat until they begin to pop and smoke slightly, about 3 minutes. Pour into a little dish and let cool.

5 Just before serving, stir the spinach into the tortellini mixture. Pour on the remaining dressing and toss well. Sprinkle on the sesame seeds and toss again.

Quick TORTELLINI AND GREEN BEAN SALAD WITH TOMATO PESTO

*I am exceptionally fond of the tomato pesto sauce that dresses hot capellini in my second book, **Quick Vegetarian Pleasures**, and I have found a wonderful way to adapt it to this cold tortellini salad. Paired with bright, crunchy green beans, this becomes a perfect pasta salad for a summer picnic.*

THE PESTO

½ cup good-quality tomato paste

⅓ cup olive oil

¼ cup grated Parmesan cheese

2 garlic cloves, pressed or minced

2 tablespoons pine nuts

3 tablespoons finely chopped fresh basil, or 1½ teaspoons dried basil *and* ¼ cup chopped fresh parsley

¼ teaspoon salt

Freshly ground black pepper

....

1 pound green beans, each cut in half (about 4 cups)

1 pound frozen cheese tortellini

Serves 4

1 To make the pesto, whisk the tomato paste and olive oil together in a medium-size bowl. Whisk in the cheese, garlic, pine nuts, basil, salt, and pepper. Set aside.

2 Bring a stockpot of water to a boil. Drop the green beans in and cook until tender yet slightly crunchy and still bright green, about 5 minutes. Remove with a slotted spoon and immerse in cold water to stop further cooking. Pour out the water and replace with more cold water. Remove the green beans and place on a cotton kitchen towel. Pat dry.

3 Drop the tortellini into the boiling water and cook until tender yet firm, about 5 minutes. Drain in a colander and shake out any excess water. Place in a large serving bowl.

4 Mix in the green beans. Scrape the pesto onto the mixture and toss to coat well. Serve at room temperature. The salad can be prepared up to 24 hours in advance; bring it to room temperature before serving.

SOBA SALAD

The nutty flavor of soba is delicious in a cold salad. Because both soba and tofu are delicate and break easily, you must handle them gingerly (good pun!) and not toss too much.

The soba and tofu can be prepared up to 4 hours in advance but should be kept separate until serving time.

8 ounces soba (buckwheat noodles)

½ cucumber, peeled, seeded, and julienned

1 carrot, julienned or grated

1 scallion, very thinly sliced

½ pound extra-firm tofu

3 tablespoons tamari soy sauce

2 tablespoons Oriental sesame oil

1 tablespoon mirin (sweet sake) or sherry

1 tablespoon balsamic or red wine vinegar

2 teaspoons sugar

½ teaspoon minced fresh ginger

Serves 3

1 Bring a large pot of water to a boil. Drop in the soba and cook until al dente, no longer than 5 minutes. Be certain not to overcook the soba; it should be chewy. Drain in a colander and run cold water over it, tossing gently. Shake the colander and drain very thoroughly. Place in a large serving bowl. Place the cucumber, carrot, and scallion on top of the noodles. Don't mix in yet.

2 Slice the tofu into ½-inch thick slices, then pat with a cotton towel or paper towels until very dry. Press lightly to extract as much moisture as possible. Cut the tofu into ½-inch cubes and place them in a medium-size bowl.

3 Combine the tamari, sesame oil, mirin, vinegar, sugar, and ginger in a cup. Drizzle about 1 tablespoon over the tofu and very gently toss to coat evenly. Let sit a few minutes to absorb the dressing.

4 Pour the remaining mixture on the soba and vegetables and toss gently but thoroughly. Let sit a few minutes so the sauce will be absorbed. Serve the soba on large plates with some marinated tofu placed on top.

ROTINI, ASPARAGUS, AND ALMOND SALAD WITH SESAME DRESSING

Quick

This light and flavorful salad is perfect for a summer day when you want to avoid heavy foods.

THE DRESSING

2 tablespoons tamari soy sauce

3 tablespoons Chinese rice vinegar or red wine vinegar

1½ tablespoons brown sugar

1½ tablespoons Oriental sesame oil

¼ cup vegetable or peanut oil

Liberal seasoning of freshly ground pepper

....

1 pound asparagus, bottom of stalks peeled, then cut diagonally into 1½-inch pieces

½ pound rotini (short corkscrew pasta)

4 scallions, thinly sliced

6 radishes, thinly sliced

½ cup sliced almonds, lightly toasted

Serves 4

1 Combine all the ingredients for the dressing in a screw-top jar and shake vigorously. Set aside.

2 Bring a large pot of water to a boil. Drop in the asparagus and let return to a boil. Cook until the asparagus is tender yet still slightly crunchy, about 3 minutes. Remove with a slotted spoon and immerse in cold water to stop further cooking. Drain, pat dry, then place the asparagus in a large bowl.

3 Stir the rotini into the boiling water and cook until tender yet still a little chewy, about 5 minutes. Drain thoroughly in a colander, then mix the rotini into the asparagus. Stir in the scallions, radishes, and almonds.

4 Pour on the dressing and toss. Serve at room temperature, or cover and chill up to 8 hours. Bring to room temperature before serving.

SUMMER EGGPLANT AND PENNE SALAD

▌ love to make this colorful salad at the end of summer when vegetables are plentiful and at their peak. Serve it with grilled garlic bread or baked French bread with Parmesan cheese.

1 medium (1¼ pounds) eggplant, peeled and cut into 1-inch cubes (no smaller)

6 tablespoons olive oil

2 yellow peppers, thinly sliced into strips

½ pound penne (quill-shaped pasta)

2 medium ripe tomatoes, cut into small cubes

4 garlic cloves, minced

2 scallions, very thinly sliced

1½ cups frozen peas, thawed

1 cup shredded fresh basil

2 tablespoons balsamic or red wine vinegar

1 teaspoon ground cumin

¾ teaspoon salt

Very generous seasoning of freshly ground pepper

2 cups arugula leaves, each cut in half (optional)

Serves 4 to 6 as a main course

1 Preheat the oven to 450 degrees.

2 Place the eggplant cubes in a large bowl, then pour 2 tablespoons of the olive oil over them. Toss quickly to coat evenly. Spread the eggplant cubes on a baking sheet so they rest in one layer. Bake 10 minutes, tossing a few times, or until the eggplant is tender but not at all mushy. The eggplant will continue to cook as it cools. Set aside to cool.

3 Heat 1 tablespoon of the olive oil in a large skillet over high heat. Add the peppers and sauté quickly for 2 to 3 minutes, or just until they are heated through. Scrape into a very large bowl and let cool.

4 Bring a medium-size saucepan of water to a boil. Drop in the penne and cook until tender yet chewy, about 10 minutes. Drain thoroughly in a colander, then run under cold water to cool. Drain again, shaking out as much water as you can. Stir the penne into the peppers.

5 Pour on the remaining 3 tablespoons of oil, toss, then mix in all the remaining ingredients except the arugula. Let sit 1 to 4 hours to marinate. Cover and chill if longer than 1 hour. Bring to room temperature before serving. If you are using the arugula, mix it in at serving time.

Quick CURRIED COUSCOUS SALAD WITH GINGER-LIME DRESSING

This salad has a marvelous blend of tantalizing flavors and textures, and the only cooking involved is boiling water, so it's a great choice for summer weather.

1½ cups couscous

½ cup golden raisins

2 teaspoons curry powder

2 cups boiling water

½ cup coarsely chopped roasted (unsalted) cashews

1½ cups frozen peas, thawed

1 red bell pepper, cut into small dice

⅓ cup slivered red onion

2 tablespoons finely chopped fresh mint or cilantro

THE DRESSING

⅓ cup fresh lime juice (3 limes)

½ teaspoon ground cumin

1 teaspoon minced fresh ginger

2 garlic cloves, minced

½ teaspoon salt

Generous seasoning of freshly ground pepper

⅓ cup olive oil

Serves 4

1 Place the couscous, raisins, and curry powder in a large serving bowl. Pour on the boiling water, stir, and tightly cover with foil or a large plate. Let sit 5 minutes, then fluff with a fork. Cover again and let sit 10 more minutes. Fluff again, then let the couscous sit uncovered until it has cooled to room temperature.

2 Stir in the cashews, peas, red pepper, onion, and mint.

3 Combine all the dressing ingredients in a screw-top jar. Shake vigorously, pour onto the couscous, and toss. Let the salad sit at least 30 minutes, or cover and chill up to 24 hours. Bring to room temperature before serving, then taste to correct the seasoning.

CURRIED FOUR-GRAIN SALAD

Packed with grains
yet amazingly light, this salad is equally great as
summer picnic food or as an entrée in winter
with some coarse bread alongside.

½ cup barley

½ cup wild rice or brown rice

½ cup bulghur, preferably dark, coarse-cut

½ cup couscous

1½ cups frozen peas, thawed

8 radishes, thinly sliced

2 scallions, very thinly sliced

1 cup raisins

⅓ cup chopped walnuts

1 tablespoon finely chopped cilantro or fresh parsley

THE DRESSING

¼ cup fresh lemon juice

⅓ cup olive oil

3 garlic cloves, pressed or minced

1 tablespoon curry powder

1 teaspoon salt

Liberal seasoning of freshly ground pepper

Serves 4 to 6

1 Bring about 2 quarts of water to a boil in a 3-quart saucepan. Drop in the barley and rice and cook, uncovered, for 40 minutes, or until tender when tasted. Stir occasionally. Drain thoroughly in a colander and let cool.

2 Meanwhile, place the bulghur in a medium-size bowl. Pour on boiling water to cover by 1 inch. Let sit for 25 minutes. Taste a few grains for tenderness. If they are still too hard, let sit for 5 minutes more. Place in a strainer and press out all of the liquid with the back of a spoon. Let cool.

3 Place the couscous in a medium-size bowl. Pour on ¾ cup boiling water, stir, and cover. Let sit for 10 minutes. Fluff with a fork and let cool.

4 Combine the barley, rice, bulghur, and couscous in a large bowl. Stir in the peas, radishes, scallions, raisins, walnuts, and cilantro.

5 Combine all the dressing ingredients in a screw-top jar and shake vigorously. Pour onto the salad and toss well. Let marinate at least 2 hours before serving. Chill if marinating longer. Serve at room temperature so that the grains are tender; they become firm when cold.

Quick BLACK BEAN SALAD WITH PINEAPPLE AND HOT PEPPERS

This marinated bean salad juxtaposes sweet pineapple with zesty hot peppers to make a spunky, colorful main course that is peppered with crunchy vegetables. Crusty bread and a soft cheese such as Brie or chèvre would be welcome companions to this salad entrée.

THE MARINADE

3 tablespoons fresh lime juice (1½ limes)

4 tablespoons olive oil

½ teaspoon ground cumin

2 garlic cloves, pressed

½ teaspoon crushed red pepper flakes

¼ teaspoon salt

....

4 cups cooked black beans (see note)

....

½ tablespoon olive oil

1 small red bell pepper, cored and cut into ½-inch dice

1 small green bell pepper, cored and cut into ½-inch dice

1½ cups diced (¾ inch) pineapple, fresh or canned

3 scallions, very thinly sliced

1 In a small bowl, whisk together all the ingredients for the marinade. Place the beans in a large bowl and pour half of the marinade on them. Stir occasionally to coat.

2 Heat the ½ tablespoon of oil in a skillet. Add the red and green peppers and sauté for 5 minutes, or until tender yet still quite crunchy. Spoon into a medium-size bowl and let cool completely.

3 Stir the pineapple, scallions, celery, optional cilantro, and pepper into the cooled peppers. Pour on the remaining marinade. (The beans and the vegetable mixture can be prepared and chilled up to 4 hours in advance. They should be kept separate so the beans don't discolor the vegetables. Bring to room temperature before serving.)

4 Just before serving, gently mix the vegetables into the beans. Place a bed of lettuce leaves on each plate. Remove the vegetables and beans from the marinade with a slotted spoon and mound on the lettuce leaves.

❧ *Note:* If you want to use dried beans, soak

1 celery rib, very thinly sliced

1 tablespoon finely chopped cilantro (optional)

Freshly ground pepper

Green leaf lettuce leaves for garnish

Serves 3 to 4

1½ cups dried black beans overnight. Drain. Cover with fresh water and cook 30 to 40 minutes, or until tender but not mushy. Drain and cool completely. If you want to use canned black beans, rinse and drain two 1-pound cans.

WARM LENTIL SALAD WITH WALNUTS, GREEN BEANS, AND RED ONION

The generous addition to this salad of lightly cooked red onion adds not only a deep flavor but also vibrant color. Sautéing red onion with just a splash of vinegar sets its color at a dazzling purple—a trick worth knowing for the charm it lends a dish. If timing makes it too difficult to serve this salad warm, it is also delicious at room temperature.

THE DRESSING

¼ cup olive oil

2 tablespoons red wine vinegar

½ teaspoon Dijon mustard

2 garlic cloves, pressed or minced

2 teaspoons fresh thyme, or ½ teaspoon dried

½ teaspoon salt

Liberal seasoning of freshly ground pepper

....

1 teaspoon olive oil

1 large red onion, halved vertically and thinly sliced

1 teaspoon red wine vinegar

½ pound green beans, cut into 2-inch lengths (2 cups)

1½ cups lentils

½ cup chopped walnuts

1 Combine all the ingredients for the dressing in a screw-top jar and shake vigorously. Set aside.

2 Heat the teaspoon of oil in a medium-size skillet. Add the red onion and sauté 2 minutes. To set the color, sprinkle the vinegar over the onions and toss well. Sauté about 5 more minutes, or just until they become tender yet still crunchy. Remove from the heat.

3 Bring about 6 cups of water to a boil in a 3-quart saucepan. Drop in the green beans and let the water return to a boil. Cook 5 minutes, or until tender yet still bright green. Remove the green beans with a slotted spoon and place in a medium-size bowl. Pour on about 1 tablespoon of dressing and set aside. Keep the water in the saucepan boiling.

4 Drop the lentils into the boiling water. After the water returns to a boil, cook the lentils, partially covered, for 15 to 20 minutes. Stir occasionally. The lentils are done when they are tender but still a tad crunchy. Do not let them get at all

¼ cup chopped fresh parsley

Lettuce leaves (optional)

Serves 4

mushy. Drain in a colander, then transfer to a large serving bowl. Pour on the dressing, toss well, and stir in the walnuts.

5 When the lentils are warm, not hot, stir in the green beans, red onions, and parsley. Serve as is or on a few lettuce leaves.

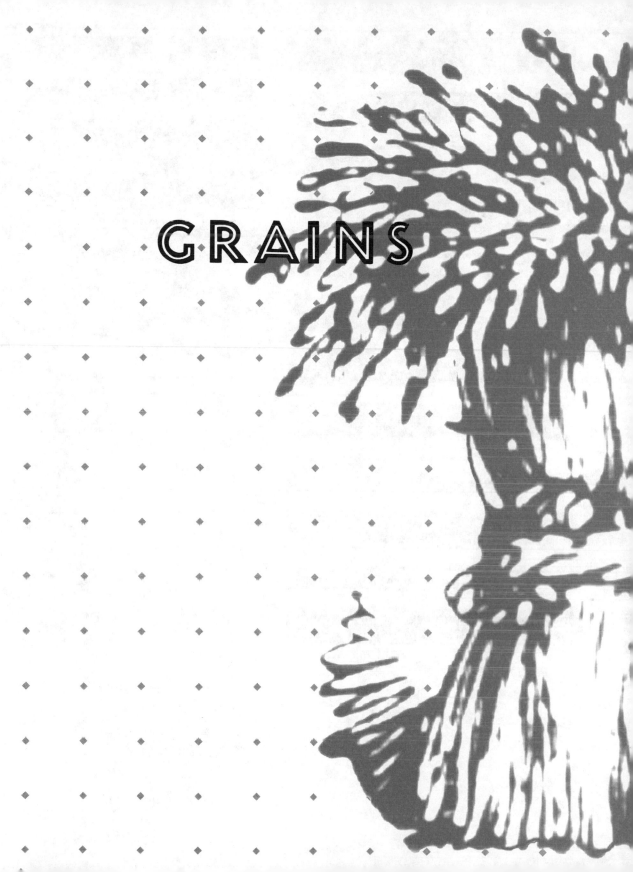

GRAINS

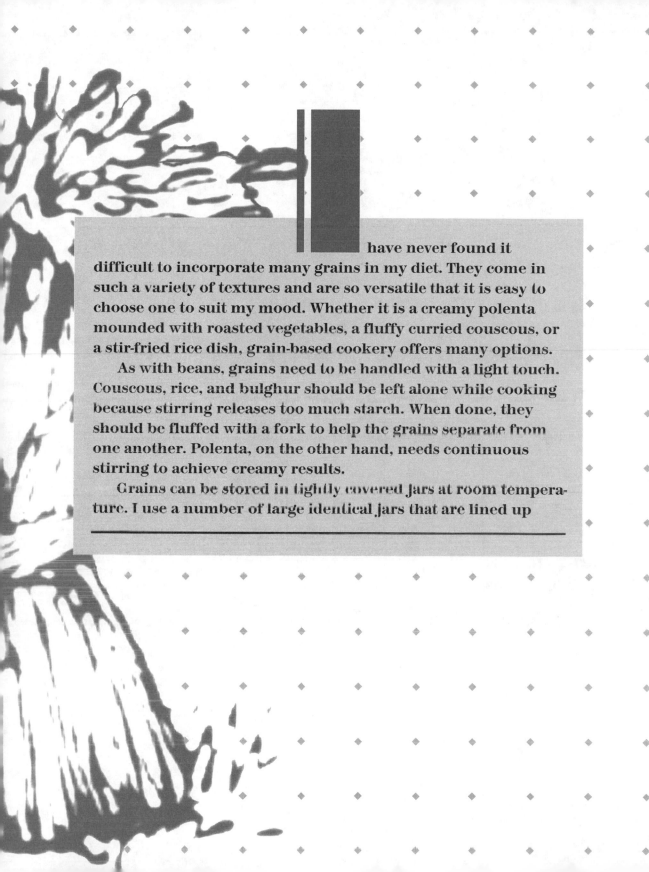

have never found it difficult to incorporate many grains in my diet. They come in such a variety of textures and are so versatile that it is easy to choose one to suit my mood. Whether it is a creamy polenta mounded with roasted vegetables, a fluffy curried couscous, or a stir-fried rice dish, grain-based cookery offers many options.

As with beans, grains need to be handled with a light touch. Couscous, rice, and bulghur should be left alone while cooking because stirring releases too much starch. When done, they should be fluffed with a fork to help the grains separate from one another. Polenta, on the other hand, needs continuous stirring to achieve creamy results.

Grains can be stored in tightly covered jars at room temperature. I use a number of large identical jars that are lined up

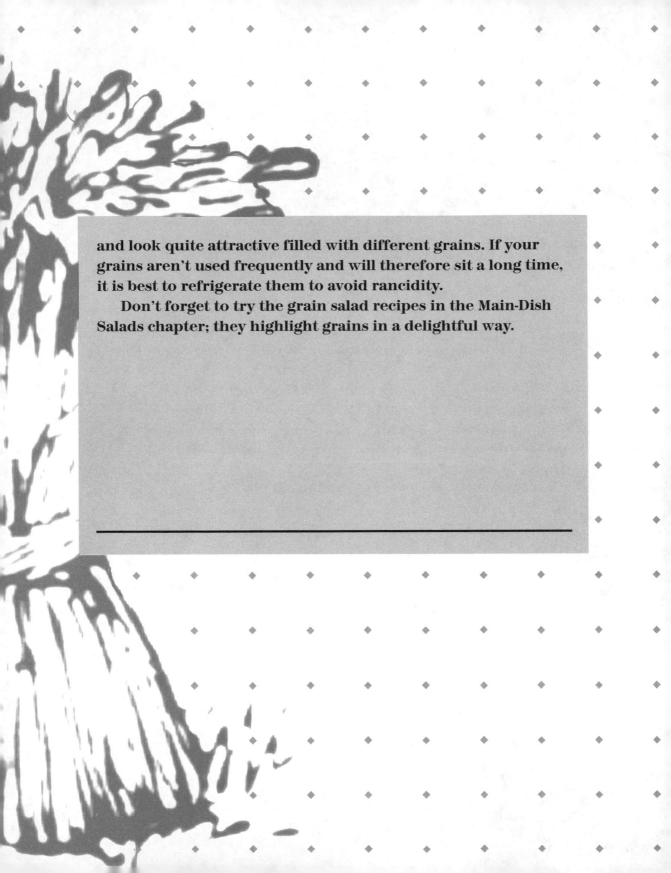

and look quite attractive filled with different grains. If your grains aren't used frequently and will therefore sit a long time, it is best to refrigerate them to avoid rancidity.

Don't forget to try the grain salad recipes in the Main-Dish Salads chapter; they highlight grains in a delightful way.

ROASTED VEGETABLES WITH POLENTA

Roasting large chunks of vegetables imparts them with a deep flavor and an alluring brown coating. Garlic cooked by this method becomes sweet and mellow, so be sure to include it.

2 small zucchini, sliced diagonally ¾-inch thick

1 red bell pepper, cored and cut into 1½-inch-square pieces

1 green bell pepper, cored and cut into 1½-inch-square pieces

1 large tomato, cored and cut into eighths

2 celery ribs, sliced diagonally ½-inch thick

8 garlic cloves, peeled

1 teaspoon dried thyme

Freshly ground pepper

3 tablespoons olive oil

2 medium onions, sliced ½-inch thick

Salt to taste

THE POLENTA

4 cups water

½ teaspoon salt

1¼ cups cornmeal

1 tablespoon butter, cut into bits

⅓ cup grated Parmesan cheese

Serves 4

1 Preheat the oven to 425 degrees.

2 Place the zucchini, peppers, tomato, celery, and garlic cloves in a large bowl. Sprinkle on the thyme and season with black pepper. Pour on two tablespoons of the oil and toss to coat. Spread the vegetable mixture onto a large baking sheet so that it is in one layer. Set aside.

3 Pour the remaining tablespoon of oil into a pie plate or 9- to 10-inch shallow pan and spread evenly. Carefully place the sliced onions in the dish, keeping them intact. Rub the bottom of the onions in the oil to coat them, then turn each slice over. Place the vegetables and onions in the oven and cook 25 to 30 minutes. Remove after 15 minutes and turn the vegetables and onions over with tongs. They are done when tender and brown. Season the vegetables with salt. Let cool while making the polenta because the vegetables are more flavorful served warm, not piping hot.

4 To make the polenta, bring the water and salt to a boil in a medium-size saucepan. Reduce the heat to medium and slowly drizzle in the cornmeal, whisking all the while. Continue to whisk until the polenta is thick and begins to tear away from the sides of the pan, about 7 minutes. Stir in the butter and cheese. Serve some polenta on each plate and top with the roasted vegetables.

BROCCOLI RABE WITH TOMATO-CHEESE POLENTA

Quick

Richard Sax, in his much-treasured book From the Farmers' Market, *recommends the Sicilian trick of pairing raisins with broccoli rabe to sweeten the slight bitterness of the greens. Here, a dynamic blending of spiciness, sweetness, and mild bitterness is the backdrop for an intriguing vegetable topping for the cheesy polenta, which is interlaced with bits of tomato.*

3½ cups vegetable stock

¼ teaspoon salt

....

1 pound broccoli rabe

2 tablespoons olive oil

6 garlic cloves, minced

¼ teaspoon crushed red pepper flakes

¼ cup raisins

¼ teaspoon salt

1 tablespoon water

THE POLENTA

1¼ cups cornmeal

¼ teaspoon salt

1 tablespoon unsalted butter

3 tablespoons grated Parmesan cheese

½ cup seeded and diced canned or fresh tomatoes, well drained

Serves 3

1 In a medium-size saucepan, bring the vegetable stock and salt to a boil for the polenta. Meanwhile, chop off all but 1 inch of the broccoli rabe stems and discard. Wash the greens and coarsely chop them. You should get about 8 cups.

2 Heat the oil in a large skillet over medium-high heat. Add the garlic and red pepper flakes and sauté 2 minutes. Do not let the garlic brown.

3 Add the broccoli rabe, raisins, salt, and water. Toss well, then cover the pan. Cook 3 to 5 minutes, or until the broccoli rabe wilts yet still retains some crunch. Remove the cover and keep warm.

4 When the vegetable stock boils, reduce the heat to a simmer. Very slowly drizzle in the cornmeal, whisking all the while. Continue to whisk until the polenta thickens and begins to pull away from the sides of the pan, about 5 minutes.

5 Remove from the heat, then whisk in the salt, butter, and Parmesan cheese. Very gently stir in the tomatoes. Serve a generous portion of polenta on each plate and top with the broccoli rabe mixture.

Quick POLENTA AND GORGONZOLA "PIZZA"

This polenta dish cuts like a pie and the slices nicely retain their shape. Topped with mozzarella cheese, tomato slices, and crumbled blue cheese, these hearty wedges need just a salad to accompany them—perhaps one made with arugula and other greens.

3 cups water

½ teaspoon salt

⅛ teaspoon grated nutmeg

1 cup cornmeal

1 tablespoon unsalted butter

¼ cup grated Parmesan cheese

1 cup (3 ounces) grated part-skim mozzarella

1 medium-size tomato, cored and thinly sliced

½ cup (about 2 ounces) crumbled Gorgonzola or other blue cheese

Freshly ground pepper

Serves 4 to 6

1 Butter a 9-inch pie plate and keep near the stove.

2 In a 2½- to 3-quart saucepan, bring the water, salt, and nutmeg to a boil. Reduce the heat to low and then drizzle in the cornmeal, whisking all the while to prevent clumping. Cook about 5 minutes, constantly whisking, or until the polenta begins to pull away from the sides of the pan.

3 Remove from the heat and whisk in the butter and Parmesan cheese. With a rubber spatula, scrape the polenta into the baking dish, smoothing the top. Let sit 10 minutes, or cover and chill up to 4 hours. Bring to room temperature before beginning step 5

4 Preheat the oven to 400 degrees.

5 Cover the top of the polenta with the grated mozzarella. Lay the tomato slices over the cheese. Sprinkle the Gorgonzola over the tomatoes, then season with the pepper

6 Bake 20 minutes, or until hot and sizzling. Cut into wedges.

Quick POLENTA WITH CAULIFLOWER, TOMATOES, AND HOT PEPPERS

The trio of tomatoes, garlic, and hot peppers is a natural match for cauliflower, highlighting its delicate flavor. When paired with polenta, this becomes a noteworthy dish.

1 tablespoon olive oil

6 garlic cloves, minced

¼ teaspoon crushed red pepper flakes

1½ cups finely chopped canned tomatoes, with their juice

1 medium (2 pounds) cauliflower, cut into small florets

· ·

4 cups vegetable stock

¼ teaspoon salt

1¼ cups cornmeal

1 tablespoon unsalted butter

⅓ cup grated Parmesan cheese

¼ cup minced fresh parsley

Serves 4

1 Heat the oil in a large skillet over medium heat. Add the garlic and pepper flakes and sauté for 2 minutes. Stir in the tomatoes and simmer for 5 minutes.

2 Mix in the cauliflower and toss to coat thoroughly with the sauce. Cover the pan and cook 5 minutes. Remove the cover, then continue to cook the cauliflower, tossing occasionally, until it is tender and the juices have thickened slightly, about 5 more minutes.

3 Meanwhile, bring the vegetable stock and salt to a boil. Very slowly drizzle in the cornmeal, whisking continuously with a wire whisk. Immediately reduce the heat to low; continue whisking the polenta until it is thick like mashed potatoes, about 5 minutes. Whisk in the butter and Parmesan cheese.

4 Stir the parsley into the cauliflower mixture. Serve the polenta on the center of each plate with a mound of cauliflower on top of it.

CORN AND SCALLION SPOONBREAD

Spoonbread is a cross between polenta and a corn soufflé, and it's best eaten with a spoon. For a harmonious side dish, try some sautéed broccoli or kale with a good dose of garlic.

3 cups low-fat milk

½ teaspoon salt

1¼ cups cornmeal

4 tablespoons unsalted butter, cut into pieces

3 eggs, separated

1½ teaspoons baking powder

1 cup frozen corn kernels, thawed

2 scallions, very thinly sliced

Serves 4

1 Butter a deep 2-quart baking dish or soufflé dish and set aside.

2 Bring 2½ cups of the milk and the salt to a boil in a medium-size saucepan. Reduce to a simmer, then slowly sprinkle in the cornmeal, whisking all the while. Cook about 5 minutes, whisking constantly. It will be thick. Whisk in the butter, then scrape into a large bowl. Let cool.

3 Preheat the oven to 350 degrees.

4 Beat the egg yolks into the cornmeal mixture. Combine the remaining ½ cup of milk with the baking powder, then beat it in.

5 Whip the egg whites until they hold stiff peaks. Spoon them onto the cornmeal mixture, then gently fold them in.

6 Pour half the batter into the prepared baking dish. Sprinkle on the corn and scallions. Top with the remaining batter. Bake 60 minutes, or until a knife inserted in the center comes out clean. Serve immediately.

Quick COUSCOUS WITH PROVENÇAL VEGETABLES

A delicious vegetable concoction with green beans, tomatoes, red peppers, olives, pine nuts, and basil is mounded on a bed of couscous to make a light but intensely flavored dish. French bread is all you need to round off the meal.

2 tablespoons olive oil

3 garlic cloves, minced

¼ teaspoon crushed red pepper flakes

1½ cups finely chopped canned tomatoes with their juice

½ pound green beans, cut diagonally into 1½-inch lengths (3 cups)

1 red bell pepper, cored and cut into 1-inch dice

....

1½ cups vegetable stock

¼ teaspoon salt

1 cup couscous

1 tablespoon unsalted butter, cut into bits

....

10 kalamata olives, pitted and coarsely chopped (see note, page 25)

2 tablespoons pine nuts

2 tablespoons minced fresh basil

Serves 3

1 Heat the oil in a large skillet over medium heat. Sauté the garlic and red pepper flakes for 1 minute, then stir in the tomatoes and their juice. Bring to a boil, mix in the green beans and red bell pepper, then cover the pan. Cook, stirring occasionally, until the green beans are tender, 10 to 15 minutes.

2 Meanwhile, make the couscous. Bring the vegetable stock and salt to a boil in a medium-size saucepan. Stir in the couscous, cover the pan, and remove from the heat. Let sit 5 minutes, or until all the stock is absorbed. Fluff with a fork, then stir in the butter. Cover again and let sit until ready to serve.

3 When the green beans are tender, check to see that there is enough liquid to make a sauce. If not, stir in a few tablespoons of water. Mix in the olives, pine nuts, and basil. Serve a bed of couscous on each plate and top with a mound of the vegetable mixture.

Quick SKILLET CURRIED VEGETABLES AND COUSCOUS WITH ALMONDS

Everything is cooked together in one pan, which makes this colorful dish a snap to prepare.

2 tablespoons unsalted butter

2 garlic cloves, minced

2 teaspoons minced fresh ginger

4 teaspoons curry powder

Dash of cayenne (or more to taste)

1 red bell pepper, cored and cut into ½-inch dice

1 carrot, very thinly sliced

2 cups tiny broccoli florets

1 small apple, peeled, cored, and cut into ½-inch dice

2 scallions, thinly sliced

½ cup frozen peas, thawed

¼ cup raisins

¼ cup sliced almonds

2½ cups vegetable stock

1½ cups couscous

½ teaspoon salt

Serves 3 to 4

1 Melt the butter in a large skillet over medium heat. Add the garlic, ginger, curry powder, and cayenne and sauté for 1 minute. Stir in the red pepper, carrot, broccoli, and ¼ cup of water. Cover the pan and steam the vegetables until almost tender, about 3 minutes.

2 Mix in the apple, scallions, peas, raisins, and almonds. Pour in the stock and bring to a boil. Stir in the couscous and salt, cover the pan, and remove it from the heat. Let sit for 7 minutes. Remove the cover, fluff the couscous with a fork, then cover again. Let sit 2 more minutes before serving.

MIXED GREENS WITH GARLIC ON COUSCOUS

Quick

I love to combine
kale with escarole in this dish, but feel free to
substitute other fresh greens, such as spinach,
broccoli rabe, collards, or mustard greens.

2 pounds fresh greens
(weight with stems), such
as kale, escarole, or
spinach

2 tablespoons olive oil

6 garlic cloves, minced

¼ teaspoon crushed red
pepper flakes

Salt

....

1½ cups vegetable stock

¼ teaspoon salt

1 cup couscous

Serves 3

1 Remove the coarse stems from the greens and discard. Thicker greens such as kale and collards will take longer to cook, so if you are using those greens in combination with more delicate greens, keep them separate. Wash the greens by dunking them in a large pot of cold water. Place the greens in a colander; discard the water. Repeat until no sand remains on the bottom of the pot.

2 Place the thicker greens in the pot with only the water that clings to them. Cover and cook over medium heat just until they begin to wilt. Add the more delicate, quicker-cooking greens, cover the pot, and cook quickly, until everything is wilted. Drain in a colander, pressing out excess liquid with the back of a spoon.

3 Heat the oil in a large skillet over medium heat. Add the garlic and red pepper flakes and cook 2 minutes—do not let it brown. Add the greens, mix well, and cook until the greens are tender yet still a bright color, about 3 minutes. Season rather generously with salt.

4 To make the couscous, bring the stock and salt to a boil in a small saucepan. Pour in the couscous, cover the pot, then remove from the heat. Let sit 5 minutes, then fluff with a fork. Serve the couscous on each plate with the greens mounded in the center.

Quick MEXICAN RICE WITH VEGETABLES AND CILANTRO

I often choose this rice dish when I crave something that's low-fat and basic, yet hearty. Everything is cooked together in a large skillet, making it a breeze to prepare. Don't hesitate to make this in advance because it is actually fluffier if it cools and is then reheated. Just sprinkle on a few tablespoons of water and reheat slowly.

2 tablespoons olive oil

1 medium onion, finely diced

2 garlic cloves, minced

1 green pepper, finely diced

2 cups (½ pound) diced green beans

1½ cups converted rice

1 tablespoon chili powder

½ teaspoon salt

Generous seasoning of freshly ground pepper

3 tablespoons tomato paste

3 cups water

2 cups cooked kidney beans, either home-cooked or canned, rinsed thoroughly if canned

3 tablespoons finely chopped cilantro

½ teaspoon dried oregano

Serves 4

1 Heat the oil in a large skillet over medium-high heat. Add the onion and garlic and sauté 2 minutes. Stir in the green pepper, green beans, rice, chili powder, salt, and pepper and, tossing often, cook 2 minutes.

2 Combine the tomato paste with about ½ cup of the water and stir to thin out the tomato paste. Stir in the remaining water and mix well. Pour into the skillet and cover the pan. Bring to a boil, then reduce to a simmer. Cook 20 minutes, or until all the liquid is absorbed.

3 Remove from the heat. Gently stir in the kidney beans, cilantro, and oregano. Cover again and let sit 5 minutes. Serve immediately or let cool, uncovered, and reheat.

SPINACH, RICE, AND FETA CHEESE GRATIN

This delicious blending of flavors is reminiscent of the filling in spanakopita—Greek spinach pie. I prefer to use white rather than brown rice in this gratin because it adds to the creamy, delicate texture.

2½ cups water

¼ teaspoon salt

1 teaspoon olive oil

1 cup basmati or converted white rice

....

2 teaspoons olive oil

1 medium-large onion, finely diced

1 red bell pepper, cored and finely diced

2 10-ounce packages frozen chopped spinach, thawed and squeezed dry

1 cup (5 ounces) finely diced feta cheese

¼ cup grated Parmesan cheese

1 tablespoon minced fresh dill, or 1 teaspoon dried

Generous seasoning of freshly ground pepper

1 egg, beaten

1 cup low-fat milk

1 tablespoon bread crumbs

1 tablespoon olive oil

Serves 4

1 To cook the rice, bring the water, salt, and oil to a boil in a medium-size saucepan. Add the rice, cover the pot, and reduce the heat to a simmer. Cook until all the water is absorbed, about 20 minutes. Spoon the rice into a large bowl and let cool.

2 Meanwhile, heat the 2 teaspoons of oil in a large skillet over medium heat. Add the onion and sauté until it begins to brown, about 10 minutes. Stir in the red pepper and cook until tender, about 7 more minutes.

3 Preheat the oven to 375 degrees. Lightly grease a 2½-quart oval gratin or other shallow baking dish.

4 Stir the onion and pepper mixture into the rice. Mix in the spinach, feta cheese, Parmesan cheese, dill, pepper, egg, and milk.

5 Spoon the rice mixture into the prepared gratin dish and smooth the top. Sprinkle on the bread crumbs, then drizzle on the olive oil. Bake 30 minutes, or until bubbling on the edges and golden on the top.

VEGETABLE FRIED RICE

This tasty rendition of the traditional Chinese dish is filled with vegetables and bits of fried tofu. Don't omit the sesame oil because it is indispensable for flavorful fried rice. Also, be certain to cook the rice well in advance—even the night before—to make sure it is cold when you begin stir-frying.

1½ cups long-grain brown rice

3 cups water

1 teaspoon vegetable oil

½ teaspoon salt

....

2 tablespoons vegetable oil

½ pound extra-firm tofu, cut into ½-inch dice and patted very dry

3 celery ribs, thinly sliced

¼ pound (about 20) snow peas, de-strung and cut diagonally into thirds, *or* 2 cups shredded cabbage

1 carrot, grated

3 scallions, thinly sliced

¼ cup tamari soy sauce

1 tablespoon Oriental sesame oil

Serves 3 generously

1 Combine the rice, water, oil, and salt in a medium-size saucepan. Cover and bring to a boil. Reduce the heat to a simmer; cook, undisturbed, until all the water is absorbed, about 45 minutes. Spoon the rice onto a large platter or shallow dish and let cool. Cover and refrigerate until cold, at least 2 hours.

2 Heat the oil in a large skillet or wok over medium-high heat until it is hot but not smoking. Add the tofu and stir-fry until golden, about 5 minutes. Spoon onto a plate, leaving any oil behind; set aside.

3 Add the celery, snow peas, and carrot to the skillet and stir-fry 2 minutes, or just until hot. Reduce the heat to low, then stir in the tofu, rice, and scallions. Pour on the tamari and sesame oil and toss well. Cook slowly, tossing frequently, until hot throughout, about 10 minutes.

Note: You can make this fried rice in advance with very successful results. Just undercook the vegetables and when it is time to reheat, sprinkle a few tablespoons of water on the rice mixture to create steam while reheating.

TRICOLOR PEPPERS
AND RICE WITH FRESH BASIL

This peasant-style rice dish, studded with mozzarella, is a feast for the senses. Bursting with color, this low-fat sauté would be an ideal summer dish when peppers and fresh basil are in abundance. Start your rice early in the day or the night before so it is cold before you add it to the vegetables; this ensures fluffy results.

1 cup long-grain brown rice, rinsed

2 cups vegetable stock or water

1 teaspoon vegetable oil

½ teaspoon salt

....

1 tablespoon olive oil

4 garlic cloves, minced

1 green bell pepper, cored and cut into ¼ × 2-inch strips

1 red bell pepper, cored and cut into ¼ × 2-inch strips

1 yellow bell pepper, cored and cut into ¼ × 2-inch strips

2 scallions, thinly sliced

10 French oil-cured olives, pitted and halved (see note, page 25)

2 tablespoons water

½ cup chopped fresh basil

½ cup (2 ounces) very finely diced part-skim

1 Combine the rice, stock, vegetable oil, and salt in a medium-size saucepan. Cover and bring to a boil; reduce the heat to a simmer. Cook, covered, until all the water is absorbed, about 45 minutes. Gently spoon the rice into a shallow dish and let cool. Refrigerate until cold, about 2 hours.

2 Heat the olive oil in a large skillet over medium-high heat. Add the garlic and cook 1 minute. Do not let it brown. Stir in the three peppers and sauté until very tender, about 10 minutes.

3 Reduce the heat to medium. Stir in the cold rice, scallions, and olives and toss well. Sprinkle on the water and cover the pan. Cook a few minutes until the rice gets piping hot. Remove the cover and stir in the basil, mozzarella, Parmesan cheese, salt to taste, and pepper. Let cook 1 more minute. Serve immediately.

mozzarella cheese

2 tablespoons grated
Parmesan cheese

Salt

Generous seasoning of
freshly ground pepper

Serves 3

MOCK VEGETABLE RISOTTO

When I want a special main-course rice dish but don't have the time to labor over a traditional risotto, I use this short-cut method to obtain a rich and creamy rice that is filled with colorful vegetables and has its own cheese "sauce." A light salad is all you need to make it a meal.

1 tablespoon unsalted butter

1 medium onion, minced

1 cup converted white rice

2¼ cups vegetable stock

½ teaspoon salt

·······································

2 tablespoons olive oil

2 garlic cloves, minced

1 red bell pepper, cored and finely diced

1 medium zucchini, cut lengthwise into sixths and thinly sliced

¼ teaspoon fennel seeds, crushed

½ cup seeded, diced tomato, either fresh or canned

½ cup frozen peas, thawed

Liberal seasoning of freshly ground pepper

·······································

2 tablespoons white wine or dry vermouth

½ cup grated Parmesan cheese

1 Heat the butter in a 3- to 4-quart saucepan over medium heat. Add the onion and sauté for 5 minutes. Stir in the rice and sauté for 2 minutes, stirring often. Pour in the vegetable stock and salt and cover the pan. Bring to a boil, then reduce the heat to a simmer.

2 Meanwhile, heat the olive oil in a large skillet over medium-high heat. Add the garlic and cook 1 minute. Do not let it brown. Stir in the red pepper and sauté 3 minutes. Add the zucchini and fennel and cook 5 minutes, stirring often. Add the tomato and sauté 2 minutes. Stir in the peas and a generous seasoning of freshly ground pepper. Remove the pan from the heat.

3 After the rice has cooked about 17 minutes, it should be tender, not mushy, and there should be a little stock left over that has not been absorbed. At this point, stir in the wine and then all the sautéed vegetables.

4 Sprinkle in the two cheeses and the basil, then gently stir to incorporate them. Cook 1 minute and serve.

½ cup grated part-skim
mozzarella cheese

1 tablespoon minced fresh
basil

Serves 3 to 4

VEGETABLE PAELLA

*S*affron permeates
this low-fat paella, lending it its distinct flavor
and golden color. A good choice when you
want something light but special.

¼ teaspoon saffron

½ cup boiling water

2 tablespoons olive oil

4 garlic cloves, minced

1 red bell pepper, cored
and cut into ½-inch dice

1 10-ounce package frozen
baby lima beans, thawed

1 tomato, cored, seeded,
and finely diced

1½ cups converted white
rice

1 teaspoon paprika

2½ cups vegetable stock

½ cup dry white wine

½ teaspoon salt

1 cup frozen peas, thawed

1 6½-ounce jar marinated
artichoke hearts, drained

3 scallions, very thinly
sliced

½ cup finely chopped fresh
parsley

Serves 3 to 4

1 Place the saffron in a teacup or small bowl
and pour the boiling water over it. Cover it and let
steep 10 minutes.

2 Heat the oil in a large skillet over medium
heat. Add the garlic and sauté for 1 minute. Add
the red pepper, lima beans, and tomato; sauté,
stirring frequently, for 5 minutes.

3 Stir in the rice and paprika. Cook 2 minutes,
stirring often. Pour in the stock, wine, saffron
water, and salt and stir to blend. Cover the
pan and bring to a boil. Reduce the heat to a simmer and cook 15 to 20 minutes, or until the
liquid is absorbed.

4 Turn off the heat. Stir in the peas, artichoke
hearts, scallions, and parsley and cover the pan.
Let sit 5 minutes, or until heated through.

GREEK-STYLE BULGHUR AND VEGETABLES WITH FETA CHEESE

Many wonderful flavors
of Greek cooking permeate this dish. Hot
pita bread as an accompaniment would nicely
continue the theme.

1 cup golden bulghur (see note)

2 tablespoons olive oil

2 medium onions, finely diced

1 cup seeded, diced tomato, fresh or canned

2 medium zucchini, quartered lengthwise and thinly sliced

1 red or green bell pepper, cored and cut into ½-inch dice

1½ teaspoons dried oregano

¼ teaspoon thyme

Generous seasoning of freshly ground pepper

10 kalamata olives, pitted and quartered (see note, page 25)

1 cup (about 5 ounces) finely diced feta cheese

Salt

Serves 3 to 4

1 Rinse the bulghur in a sieve. Place it in a medium-size bowl and pour in enough boiling water to cover by 2 inches. Let sit 20 minutes, or until the bulghur is tender when a pinch of it is tasted.

2 In batches, place some bulghur in a strainer and press out as much water as possible with the back of a large spoon. Place this dry bulghur in a bowl and repeat the procedure with the rest.

3 Heat the oil in a large skillet over medium-high heat. Add the onions and sauté 10 minutes. Stir in the tomato and sauté 5 minutes.

4 Mix in the zucchini, bell pepper, oregano, thyme, and pepper and sauté, tossing often, until the vegetables are tender yet crisp, about 10 minutes.

5 Stir in the bulghur and olives. Cook a few more minutes, stirring frequently, until the mixture is piping hot. Sprinkle on the feta cheese and gently toss to combine. Cook 1 more minute, then taste for salt; it might need a bit. Serve immediately.

❧ *Note:* For this recipe I prefer the medium-grain golden bulghur to the coarse dark kind.

MIXED GRAINS BAKED WITH HERBS, VEGETABLES, AND CHEESE

Sometimes I crave grains, the heartier the better. This casserole offers four grains with varied textures and colors combined with herbs, vegetables, and cheese to make a savory, wholesome dish.

4 cups vegetable stock

½ cup barley

¼ cup wild rice

¼ cup brown rice

....

1 tablespoon olive oil

1 medium onion, diced

½ pound sliced mushrooms (3 cups)

1 cup finely chopped canned tomatoes, with their juice

Grated peel of 1 lemon (about 1 teaspoon)

½ cup sliced black olives (California-style)

½ cup chopped fresh parsley

2 teaspoons finely chopped fresh thyme, or ½ teaspoon dried

1 tablespoon finely chopped fresh basil, or ½ teaspoon dried

Generous seasoning of freshly ground pepper

1 Bring the vegetable stock to a boil in a medium-size saucepan. Add the barley and wild rice and simmer, covered, for 15 minutes. Stir in the brown rice and cook 10 more minutes. If you are going to cook the casserole immediately, pour the entire contents of the pot into a large, shallow 2½-quart baking dish, such as a 10 × 10-inch or 12 × 7 × 2-inch Pyrex dish. If you are not cooking right away, scoop out the grains with a slotted spoon and place them in the baking dish. Reserve the stock.

2 Preheat the oven to 350 degrees.

3 Heat the oil in a medium-size skillet. Add the onion and sauté 5 minutes. Stir in the mushrooms and cook until they begin to get brown and juicy, about 10 minutes. Scrape the mixture into the grains.

4 Stir in the tomatoes, lemon peel, olives, parsley, thyme, basil, and pepper. If you have separated the grains from the stock and you are now ready to bake the dish, bring the stock to a boil and pour into the casserole. Cover the dish and bake 30 minutes.

½ cup bulghur

1 cup frozen peas, thawed

1 cup (4 ounces) finely
cubed Cheddar cheese

Serves 4 to 6

5 Remove the casserole from the oven and stir in the bulghur. Cover again and return to the oven. Cook 25 more minutes, or until all the liquid has been absorbed and the grains are tender.

6 Fluff the mixture with a fork; gently stir in the peas and cheese. Cover again and let sit outside the oven for 10 minutes before serving.

GARLICKY SWISS CHARD SAUTÉ ON BULGHUR

Quick

Garlic and hot peppers team with Swiss chard and pinto beans to make an extremely tasty and nutritious topping for bulghur. Try to get young Swiss chard with slender stalks so it will be extra tender.

2 cups vegetable stock

1 cup golden bulghur (see note, page 59)

....

2 tablespoons olive oil

4 garlic cloves, minced

¼ teaspoon crushed red pepper flakes

1¼ pounds Swiss chard (with 2-inch stems), washed and coarsely chopped (12 cups)

1 16-ounce can pinto beans, rinsed and well drained

Serves 4

1 Bring the vegetable stock to a boil in a medium-size saucepan. Add the bulghur and cover the pot. Reduce the heat to a simmer and cook until all the water is absorbed, about 20 minutes.

2 Meanwhile, heat the olive oil in a large skillet over medium-high heat. Add the garlic and pepper flakes and cook 1 minute, or until the garlic begins to turn golden but not at all brown. Drop in the Swiss chard with any water that clings to it, and with 2 large spoons, carefully toss it with the garlic mixture. Cover the pan and let the Swiss chard steam until it wilts, about 7 minutes. Toss again.

3 Stir in the pinto beans and cook 1 minute more, or until heated through. It's okay if a little liquid remains in the pan; this will serve as a sauce.

4 When the bulghur has absorbed all the stock, fluff it with a fork. Remove the pan from the heat and keep covered for 5 minutes. Serve some bulghur on each plate with a mound of the Swiss chard mixture in the center.

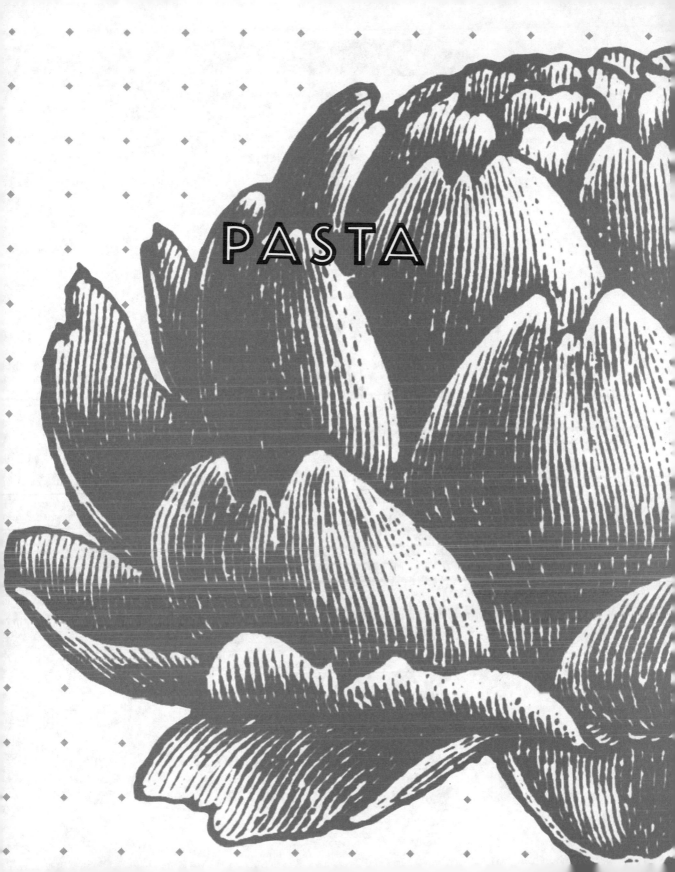

PASTA

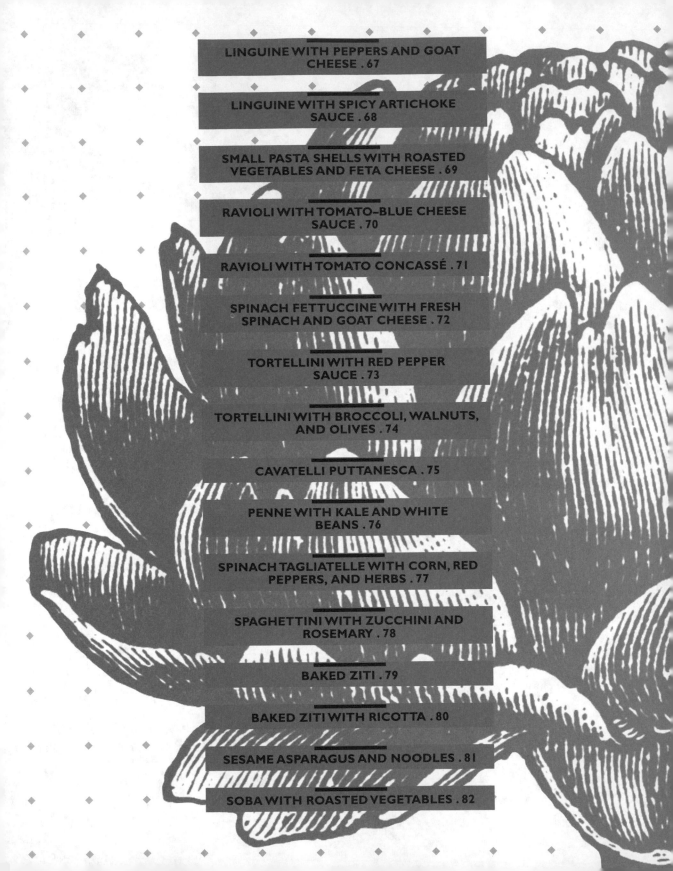

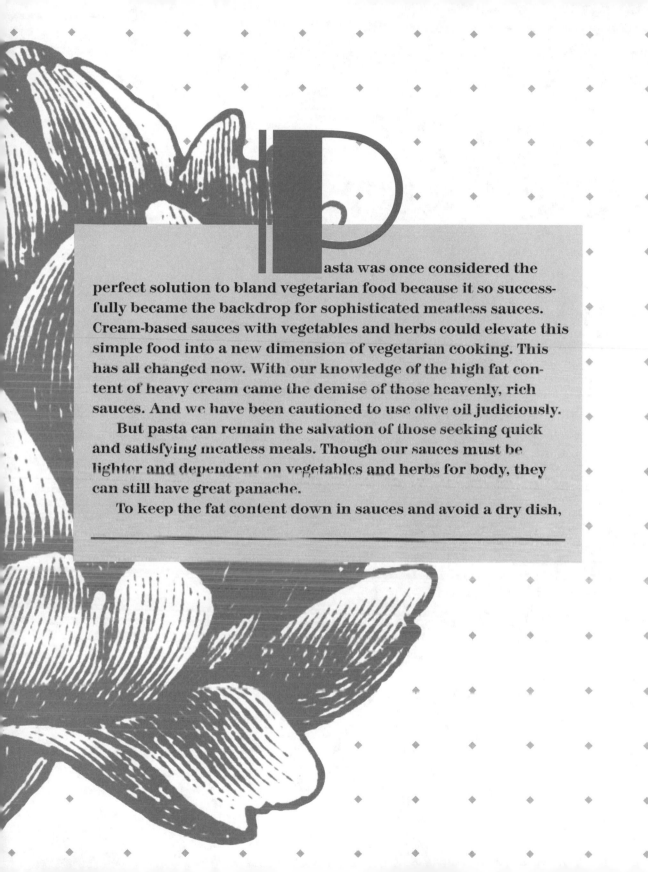

Pasta was once considered the perfect solution to bland vegetarian food because it so successfully became the backdrop for sophisticated meatless sauces. Cream-based sauces with vegetables and herbs could elevate this simple food into a new dimension of vegetarian cooking. This has all changed now. With our knowledge of the high fat content of heavy cream came the demise of those heavenly, rich sauces. And we have been cautioned to use olive oil judiciously.

But pasta can remain the salvation of those seeking quick and satisfying meatless meals. Though our sauces must be lighter and dependent on vegetables and herbs for body, they can still have great panache.

To keep the fat content down in sauces and avoid a dry dish,

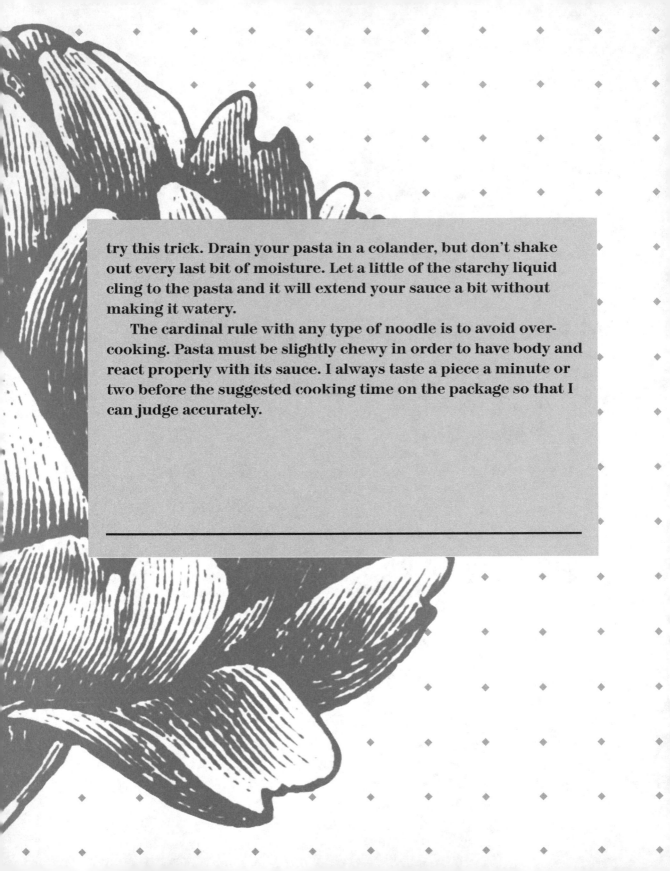

try this trick. Drain your pasta in a colander, but don't shake out every last bit of moisture. Let a little of the starchy liquid cling to the pasta and it will extend your sauce a bit without making it watery.

The cardinal rule with any type of noodle is to avoid over-cooking. Pasta must be slightly chewy in order to have body and react properly with its sauce. I always taste a piece a minute or two before the suggested cooking time on the package so that I can judge accurately.

Quick LINGUINE WITH PEPPERS AND GOAT CHEESE

This simple preparation
with goat cheese as the basis of the sauce is
especially elegant when paired with fresh pasta,
although dried pasta is also delicious. The tang
and creaminess of goat cheese in this sauce is
unmatched.

2 tablespoons olive oil

2 garlic cloves, minced

1 red bell pepper, cored
and cut into thin strips

1 green bell pepper, cored
and cut into thin strips

2 scallions, thinly sliced

¼ cup minced fresh
parsley

1 tablespoon minced fresh
basil, or 1 teaspoon dried

¼ teaspoon dried oregano

....

16 ounces fresh linguine,
or 12 ounces dried

4 ounces garlic and chive
goat cheese or plain goat
cheese, cut into small
pieces

Serves 3

1 Bring a large pot of water to a boil.

2 Meanwhile, heat the olive oil in a large skillet
over medium heat. Add the garlic and bell peppers and sauté 10 minutes, or until the peppers
are tender.

3 Add the scallions, parsley, basil, and oregano
and heat through. Keep warm while cooking the
pasta.

4 Cook the pasta in boiling water until it is al
dente. Taste a piece to avoid overcooking. Drain in
a colander. Place in a large bowl and toss with the
sauce. Sprinkle on the goat cheese and toss again.
Serve immediately.

Quick LINGUINE WITH SPICY ARTICHOKE SAUCE

Garlic, hot peppers, and the artichoke marinade bolster this spunky tomato sauce, making you want to brazenly lick your lips.

1 tablespoon olive oil

6 garlic cloves, minced

¼ teaspoon crushed red pepper flakes

1 28-ounce can plum tomatoes, finely chopped and well drained

½ teaspoon dried basil

½ teaspoon dried oregano

½ teaspoon salt

1 pound linguine

1 6-ounce jar marinated artichoke hearts

¼ cup minced fresh parsley

Grated Parmesan cheese

Serves 4

1 Heat the oil in a large skillet over medium heat. Add the garlic and pepper flakes and cook 2 minutes, tossing often. Stir in the tomatoes, basil, oregano, and salt and bring to a boil. Reduce to a simmer and cook, stirring often, for 15 minutes.

2 Meanwhile, bring a large stockpot of water to a boil. Drop in the linguine and cook until al dente. Taste a piece to avoid overcooking.

3 Add the artichokes and their marinade to the sauce. Stir in the parsley. Simmer about 5 minutes.

4 Drain the linguine and place it in a large bowl or return it to the pot. Toss with the sauce. Serve sprinkled with Parmesan cheese.

SMALL PASTA SHELLS WITH ROASTED VEGETABLES AND FETA CHEESE

This brightly colored pasta dish captures the glorious colors and seductive flavors of the Mediterranean. Garlic bread alongside adds the perfect touch.

1 small red bell pepper, cored and diced into 1-inch

1 small yellow bell pepper, cored and diced into 1-inch

1 small green bell pepper, cored and diced into 1-inch

2 tomatoes, cored, seeded, and cut into 1-inch dice

1 medium-large onion, cut into 1-inch dice, sections separated

2 celery ribs, thinly sliced on the diagonal

5 garlic cloves, coarsely chopped

1 teaspoon dried basil

1 teaspoon dried oregano

4 tablespoons olive oil

1 pound small pasta shells

1 cup (4½ ounces) finely diced feta cheese

20 black oil-cured olives, halved and pitted (see note, page 25)

Salt to taste

Generous seasoning of freshly ground pepper

Serves 4 to 6

1 Bring a large pot of water to a boil for the pasta. Preheat the oven to 425 degrees for the vegetables.

2 In a large bowl, combine the peppers, tomatoes, onion, celery, garlic, basil, oregano, and 2 tablespoons of the olive oil. Toss to coat the vegetables thoroughly with the oil. Spread the vegetables on a baking sheet so they rest in one layer. Bake for 20 minutes, or until the peppers are tender. Toss with a spatula once during baking.

3 Once the water starts boiling, drop the pasta in and cook until tender yet chewy, about 12 minutes. Drain thoroughly in a colander and either return to the pot or place it in a large bowl.

4 Spoon the vegetables onto the pasta along with the remaining 2 tablespoons of oil. Sprinkle on the feta cheese, olives, salt, and pepper (be very generous with the pepper) and toss. Serve hot or warm.

Quick RAVIOLI WITH TOMATO— BLUE CHEESE SAUCE

Uncooked sauces are a great time-saving method of dressing pasta with choice ingredients (see also Penne with Greek-Style Vegetable Marinade, page 25). This ravioli dish is best served warm, so there's no need to rush it to the table after it's been combined with the sauce.

¼ cup olive oil

1 medium-large tomato, cut into small dice

3 scallions, thinly sliced

3 tablespoons finely chopped walnuts

¼ cup finely chopped fresh parsley

Generous seasoning of freshly ground pepper

Salt to taste

....

1 pound frozen cheese ravioli

½ cup (2 ounces) crumbled blue cheese

Serves 4

1 In a large bowl, combine the oil, tomato, scallions, walnuts, parsley, pepper, and salt. Let sit for 30 minutes, or up to 4 hours. Cover and chill if longer than 1 hour, but bring to room temperature before the next step.

2 Bring a large pot of water to a boil. Drop in the ravioli and cook until tender yet still slightly firm, about 5 minutes. Drain thoroughly in a colander.

3 Toss the ravioli with the tomato mixture. Sprinkle on the blue cheese and gently toss again. Serve warm, not piping hot.

Quick RAVIOLI WITH TOMATO CONCASSÉ

Roughly chopping tomatoes and sautéing them quickly with shallots or onions makes them delightfully sweet. They serve as a tantalizing base for this simple sauce.

2 tablespoons olive oil

4 shallots, finely diced

1 16-ounce can tomatoes, finely chopped and drained

1 tablespoon minced fresh basil, or ¾ teaspoon dried

¼ teaspoon salt

Freshly ground pepper

1 pound frozen cheese ravioli

1 tablespoon butter, cut into bits

Grated Parmesan cheese

Serves 3 to 4

1 Bring a large pot of water to a boil for the ravioli.

2 Meanwhile, make the sauce. In a large skillet, heat the olive oil over medium heat. Add the shallots and sauté for 5 minutes. Add the tomatoes, basil, salt, and pepper and cook, stirring frequently, for 10 minutes.

3 Drop the ravioli into the water and cook until al dente, about 5 minutes. Drain and then add to the sauce. Toss to coat thoroughly. Add the butter bits and toss again. Serve with Parmesan cheese sprinkled on top.

Quick SPINACH FETTUCCINE WITH FRESH SPINACH AND GOAT CHEESE

The double impact of spinach pasta with fresh spinach is extremely flavorful as well as a great color combination.

1 pound loose fresh spinach, or 1 10-ounce package fresh spinach, stems discarded and leaves torn into small pieces (8 to 10 cups)

3 tablespoons olive oil

6 garlic cloves, minced

¼ teaspoon crushed red pepper flakes

1 pound spinach fettuccine

½ teaspoon salt

6 ounces goat cheese, crumbled

Serves 3 to 4

1 Bring a large pot of water to a boil for the pasta.

2 Wash the spinach in batches by dunking it in a large bowl of cold water. Remove and place in a colander.

3 Heat the oil in a large skillet over medium heat. Add the garlic and red pepper flakes and sauté 2 minutes, stirring frequently. Add the spinach with the water that clings to it and cover the pan. Cook for about 5 minutes, or until the spinach wilts.

4 Drop the fettuccine into the pot of rapidly boiling water. Cook until al dente, about 10 minutes. Remove ½ cup of the pasta water and pour it into the spinach mixture along with the salt; this will create a sauce.

5 Drain the fettuccine in a colander and return to the pot or place in a large bowl. Pour on the spinach and its liquid. Toss. Sprinkle on the goat cheese and toss again. Serve immediately.

Quick TORTELLINI WITH RED PEPPER SAUCE

Puréed red bell peppers make an extremely tasty sauce with a fiery color. For a beautiful color contrast and a nice balance of flavors, serve these tortellini with steamed, whole green beans.

THE SAUCE

1 tablespoon olive oil

1 medium onion, diced

2 garlic cloves, minced

1 large red bell pepper, cored and diced

2 fresh or canned plum tomatoes, seeded and diced

¼ cup dry red or white wine

¼ cup vegetable stock

A few dashes of cayenne

¼ teaspoon salt

1 tablespoon unsalted butter

....

1 pound frozen cheese tortellini

Grated Parmesan cheese

1 tablespoon minced fresh parsley

Serves 3

1 Bring a large pot of water to a boil for the tortellini.

2 To make the sauce, heat the oil in a medium-size skillet over medium heat. Add the onion and garlic and sauté for 5 minutes. Add the red pepper and tomatoes and cook 10 minutes more, or until the peppers are tender.

3 Pour in the wine and stock and cook at a lively simmer for 7 minutes. Purée in a blender or food processor, then return the sauce to the pan. (You should have about 1¼ cups sauce.) Stir in the cayenne, salt, and butter. Keep warm.

4 Drop the tortellini into the boiling water and cook until al dente, about 5 minutes. Drain thoroughly and return to the pot or place in a large bowl. Spoon on the sauce and toss to coat. Sprinkle on the Parmesan cheese, then top with the parsley. Serve immediately.

TORTELLINI WITH BROCCOLI, WALNUTS, AND OLIVES

This dish very nicely juxtaposes an array of flavors with the spiciness of garlic and hot peppers, the deep flavor of toasted walnuts, and the saltiness of olives. A nice choice for entertaining on a moment's notice.

¼ cup olive oil

6 garlic cloves, minced

¼ teaspoon crushed red pepper flakes

½ cup chopped walnuts

1 large bunch broccoli, cut into small florets, stalks peeled and diced (about 6 cups)

1 pound frozen cheese tortellini

12 kalamata or other brine-cured olives, pitted and quartered (see note, page 25)

¼ teaspoon salt

¼ cup grated Parmesan cheese

Serves 4

1 Bring a large pot of water to a boil.

2 To make the sauce, heat the oil in a large skillet over medium heat. Add the garlic, red pepper flakes, and walnuts. Sauté, tossing often, for 5 minutes.

3 Stir in the broccoli with ½ cup of water. Cover the pan and cook until tender yet still bright green, about 5 minutes.

4 Drop the tortellini into the boiling water and cook until tender yet firm, about 5 minutes. Drain thoroughly in a colander.

5 Mix the tortellini into the broccoli sauce along with the olives, salt, and Parmesan cheese. Serve immediately.

Quick CAVATELLI PUTTANESCA

Spicy and bold, this sauce is worthy of its name—puttanesca means "whore-style." Try it also with cheese ravioli for a nice match.

2 tablespoons olive oil

6 garlic cloves, minced

¼ teaspoon crushed red pepper flakes

1 green pepper, finely diced

1 28-ounce can whole tomatoes, drained and finely chopped with their own juice

8 black olives (preferably kalamata), pitted and quartered (see note, page 25)

2 teaspoons capers

Freshly ground pepper

1 pound frozen cavatelli

Grated Parmesan cheese (optional)

Serves 3 to 4

1 Bring a large pot of water to a boil.

2 Heat the olive oil in a large skillet over medium heat. Add the garlic and red pepper flakes and cook 2 minutes, stirring often. Add the green pepper and cook 5 minutes.

3 Stir in the tomatoes, olives, capers, and ground pepper and cook 15 to 20 minutes, or until the sauce has thickened and the green pepper is very tender.

4 Cook the cavatelli according to the package directions. Drain thoroughly in a colander, then return it to the pot or place in a large bowl. Stir in the sauce. Serve with a little Parmesan cheese, if desired; it won't need much.

Quick PENNE WITH KALE AND WHITE BEANS

The kale and white beans dominate this garlicky dish in which pasta plays only a supportive role. If you are not acquainted with kale, here's a great opportunity to discover this wonderful vegetable. It's packed with vitamin A, has a delicious flavor, and is a breeze to prepare.

1½ pounds kale

3 tablespoons olive oil

6 garlic cloves, minced

¼ teaspoon crushed red pepper flakes

⅓ cup vegetable stock

1 16-ounce can cannellini beans, rinsed and drained

½ teaspoon salt

½ pound penne (quill-shaped pasta)

¼ cup grated Parmesan cheese

Serves 3 to 4

1 Bring 3 quarts of water to a boil in a saucepan.

2 Prepare the kale by ripping it off its stems. Tear the leaves into bite-size pieces. You should have about 12 cups. Rinse by immersing in a large bowl of cold water. Remove and drain in a colander.

3 Heat the oil in a large skillet over medium-high heat. Add the garlic and red pepper flakes and sauté for 2 minutes. Stir in the kale and vegetable stock and cover the pan. Cook until wilted and tender yet still bright green, about 7 minutes. Gently stir in the beans and salt and keep warm over low heat.

4 Drop the penne into the boiling water and cook until tender yet chewy, about 10 minutes. Drain thoroughly, then carefully stir it into the kale mixture along with the Parmesan cheese. Serve immediately.

Quick SPINACH TAGLIATELLE WITH CORN, RED PEPPERS, AND HERBS

The natural sweetness of corn pairs wonderfully with the red peppers and spicy herb blend, giving this dish a charming Southwestern touch and a great splash of color.

¼ cup olive oil

1 red bell pepper, cored and cut into thin strips

¼ teaspoon crushed red pepper flakes

4 scallions, thinly sliced

2 cups frozen corn kernels, thawed

1 teaspoon dried oregano

1 tablespoon minced fresh basil, or ½ teaspoon dried

2 tablespoons minced fresh parsley

½ teaspoon salt

....

1 pound spinach tagliatelle (or spinach fettuccine)

¼ cup grated Parmesan cheese

Serves 4

1 Bring a large pot of water to a boil.

2 Heat the oil in a large skillet over medium heat. Add the red pepper and crushed pepper flakes and sauté for 5 minutes, or until just about tender. Add the scallions and cook 2 minutes, stirring occasionally. Mix in the corn, herbs, and salt. Keep warm over low heat.

3 Drop the tagliatelle into boiling water. Cook until tender yet chewy, about 7 minutes. Remove ½ cup of the pasta water and stir it into the vegetable mixture.

4 Drain the pasta. Return it to the pot or place in a large bowl. Spoon on the sauce and sprinkle on the cheese. Toss and serve immediately.

SPAGHETTINI WITH ZUCCHINI AND ROSEMARY

osemary gives this savory pasta sauce a distinct, yet not over- powering, flavor. Garlic bread is the perfect accompaniment.

2 tablespoons olive oil

2 medium onions, diced

4 medium zucchini, halved lengthwise and thinly sliced

1 teaspoon chopped fresh rosemary, or ¼ teaspoon dried, crumbled

½ teaspoon salt

Very generous seasoning of freshly ground pepper (about 20 turns of the peppermill)

1 pound spaghettini

½ cup grated Parmesan cheese

Serves 4

1 Bring a large pot of water to a boil.

2 To make the sauce, heat the olive oil in a large skillet over medium-high heat. Add the onions and sauté for 10 minutes, or until tender.

3 Mix in the zucchini, rosemary, salt, and pepper. Sauté, tossing often, until the zucchini is tender but not mushy, about 10 minutes. Keep warm over low heat.

4 Drop the pasta into the boiling water and cook until al dente. Remove ½ cup of the boiling pasta water and stir it into the zucchini mixture. Drain the spaghettini very well in a colander.

5 Place the spaghettini in a large bowl or return it to the pot. Spoon on the zucchini sauce and sprin- kle on the Parmesan cheese. Toss to coat. Serve immediately.

Quick BAKED ZITI

ere's a quick and hearty dish that I love to assemble on a moment's notice because I always seem to have these ingredients on hand. This is my idea of comfort food.

1 pound ziti or penne

2 tablespoons olive oil

1½ cups tomato sauce (homemade or store-bought)

½ teaspoon dried basil

½ teaspoon oregano

2 tablespoons dry red wine

Freshly ground pepper to taste

2 cups (6 ounces) grated Muenster cheese

¼ cup grated Parmesan cheese

Serves 6

1 Cook the ziti in a large pot of boiling water until al dente, 12 to 15 minutes. Drain thoroughly in a colander and place in a large bowl. Pour on the olive oil and toss to coat well. Let cool.

2 Combine the tomato sauce, basil, oregano, red wine, and pepper. Pour onto the pasta and mix well.

3 Preheat the oven to 350 degrees.

4 Spread half the pasta in a large, shallow baking dish, such as a 9 × 13-inch (3-quart) Pyrex. Sprinkle on half the Muenster cheese. Spread on the remaining pasta, then top with the remaining Muenster cheese and finally the Parmesan cheese. Cover the dish with foil.

5 Bake for 30 to 40 minutes, or until hot and bubbly. Remove foil and bake 5 additional minutes.

Note: The dish may be prepared in advance through step 4 and refrigerated for up to 8 hours. Bring to room temperature before baking.

Quick BAKED ZITI WITH RICOTTA

This stick-to-your-ribs version of baked ziti is reminiscent of lasagne. A good choice to serve a crowd.

1 pound ziti or penne

1½ cups tomato sauce (homemade or store-bought)

1 egg

1 15-ounce container part-skim ricotta cheese

2½ cups (8 ounces) grated part-skim mozzarella cheese

¼ cup grated Parmesan cheese

Serves 6

1 Bring a large pot of water to a boil. Cook the ziti until al dente, 12 to 15 minutes. Drain thoroughly in a colander, then place in a large bowl. Pour on the tomato sauce to coat well. Let cool.

2 Beat the egg in a medium-size bowl. Beat in the ricotta cheese and 2¼ cups of the mozzarella.

3 Preheat the oven to 400 degrees.

4 Spread half the ziti in a 9 × 13-inch (3-quart) baking dish. Spread the ricotta mixture evenly on top. Spoon on the remaining ziti, sprinkle on the reserved ¼ cup of mozzarella, then finish with the Parmesan cheese. Cover the dish with foil.

5 Bake 40 to 45 minutes, or until hot and bubbly. Remove the foil and bake 5 additional minutes.

Note: The dish may be prepared in advance through step 4 and refrigerated for up to 8 hours. Bring to room temperature before baking.

Quick SESAME ASPARAGUS AND NOODLES

Assemble all the ingredients for this tasty dish before you begin cooking and it will be a breeze to prepare.

2 tablespoons sesame seeds

....

2 tablespoons Oriental sesame oil

¼ cup tamari soy sauce

2 tablespoons vegetable stock

2 tablespoons Chinese rice wine or dry sherry

½ teaspoon chili oil

1 pound linguine or vermicelli

....

1 tablespoon vegetable oil

2 garlic cloves, minced

1 teaspoon minced fresh ginger

1 pound asparagus, cut diagonally into 2-inch lengths

¼ cup water

1 teaspoon tamari soy sauce

4 scallions, thinly sliced

Serves 3 to 4

1 Bring a large pot of water to a boil for the noodles.

2 Toast the sesame seeds by placing them in a small skillet over medium heat. Swirl the pan occasionally until the seeds begin to smoke and become fragrant. Immediately pour them into a small bowl to cool.

3 Combine the sesame oil, tamari, vegetable stock, wine, and chili oil in a measuring cup and set aside. This will be the sauce for the noodles.

4 When the water is at a rolling boil, cook the noodles until tender yet chewy.

5 Heat the vegetable oil in a large skillet or wok over medium-high heat. Add the garlic and ginger and cook 1 minute. Add the asparagus and stir-fry 1 minute. Pour in the water and cover the pan. Cook until the asparagus pieces are tender, about 5 minutes.

6 Drain the noodles and return them to the pot. Pour on the prepared sauce and toss with tongs to coat.

7 Remove the cover from the asparagus. Pour on the teaspoon of tamari and the scallions and toss for 1 minute. Serve on the noodles.

SOBA WITH ROASTED VEGETABLES

Roasted root vegetables caramelize and develop a marvelous taste as well as texture. When paired with soba, a full-flavored dish is created that also maintains the characteristic lightness of Japanese cooking. Hauntingly good.

2 tablespoons vegetable oil

1 tablespoon tamari soy sauce

2 purple-top turnips (about ¼ pound each), peeled, halved, and cut into ¾-inch slices

1 large (¾ pound) sweet potato, peeled, halved lengthwise, and cut into ½-inch slices

2 carrots, peeled, cut in half crosswise, thick top part cut in half lengthwise

2 medium onions, peeled and quartered lengthwise with root intact

8 ounces soba (buckwheat noodles)

½ cup vegetable stock

1 tablespoon tamari soy sauce

1 tablespoon Oriental sesame oil

Sesame seeds (optional garnish)

Serves 2

1 Combine the oil and tamari in a large bowl. Mix in the vegetables and toss to coat them thoroughly. Marinate for at least 30 minutes, or up to 2 hours.

2 Preheat the oven to 400 degrees.

3 Spread the vegetables on a baking sheet so they rest in one layer. Bake, tossing twice, for 25 to 30 minutes, or until the vegetables are tender.

4 Meanwhile, bring water to a boil in a 3-quart pot. Cook the soba until tender yet chewy, about 5 minutes.

5 While the soba is cooking, combine the vegetable stock, tamari, and sesame oil. Drain the soba and return to the pot. Pour on the liquid and toss gently. Serve the soba immediately in large bowls with the vegetables on top. If desired, garnish with a few sesame seeds.

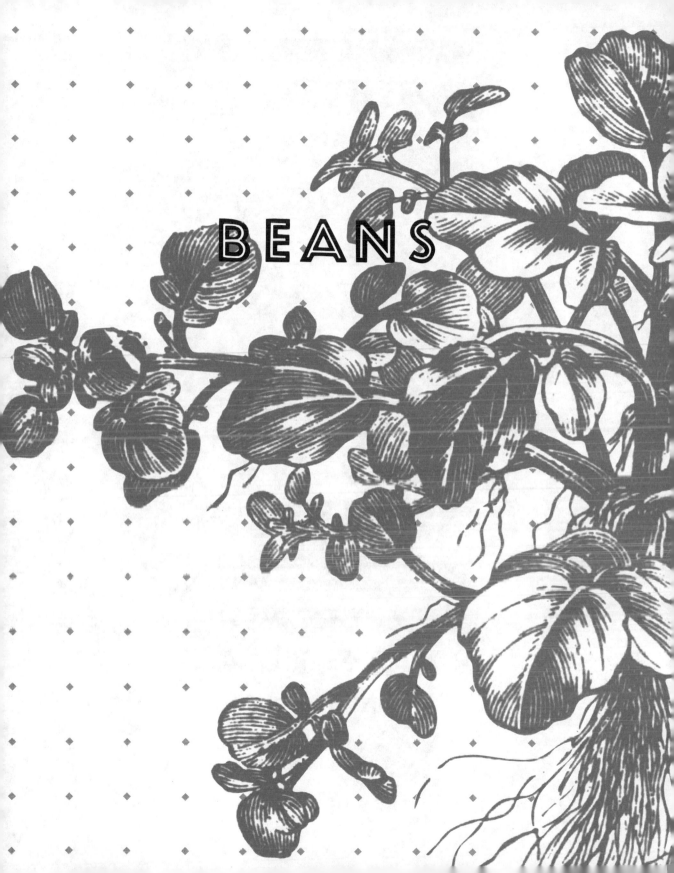

BEANS

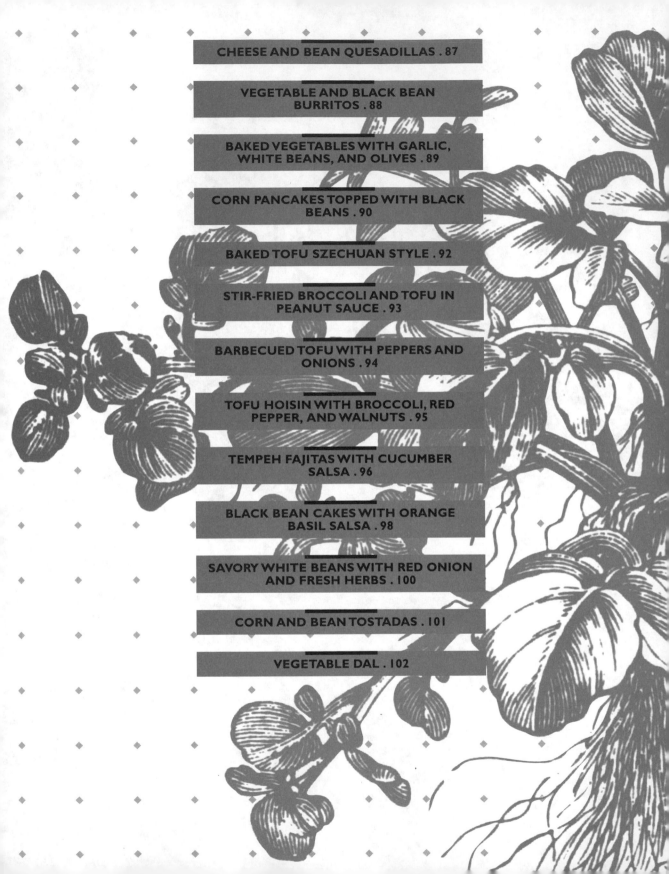

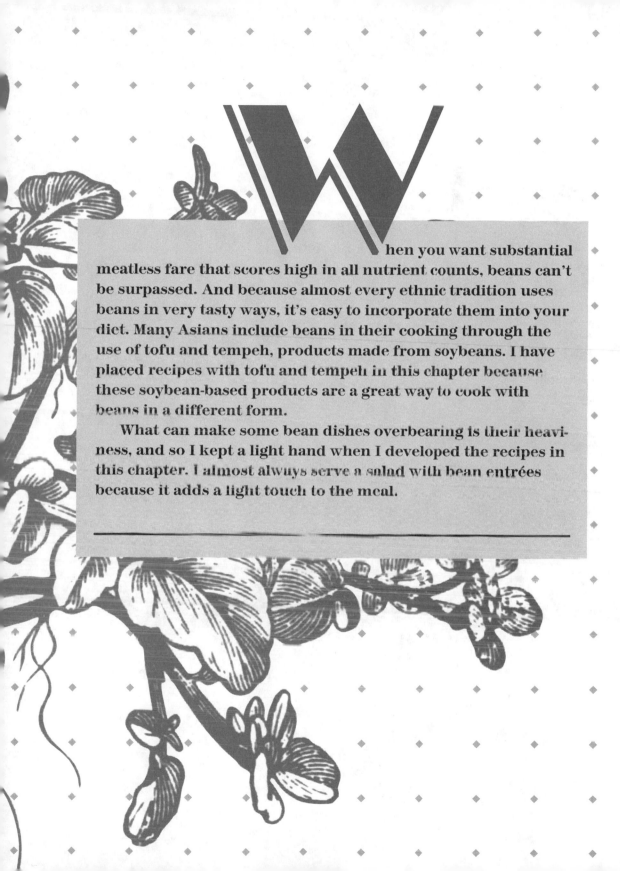

When you want substantial meatless fare that scores high in all nutrient counts, beans can't be surpassed. And because almost every ethnic tradition uses beans in very tasty ways, it's easy to incorporate them into your diet. Many Asians include beans in their cooking through the use of tofu and tempeh, products made from soybeans. I have placed recipes with tofu and tempeh in this chapter because these soybean-based products are a great way to cook with beans in a different form.

What can make some bean dishes overbearing is their heaviness, and so I kept a light hand when I developed the recipes in this chapter. I almost always serve a salad with bean entrées because it adds a light touch to the meal.

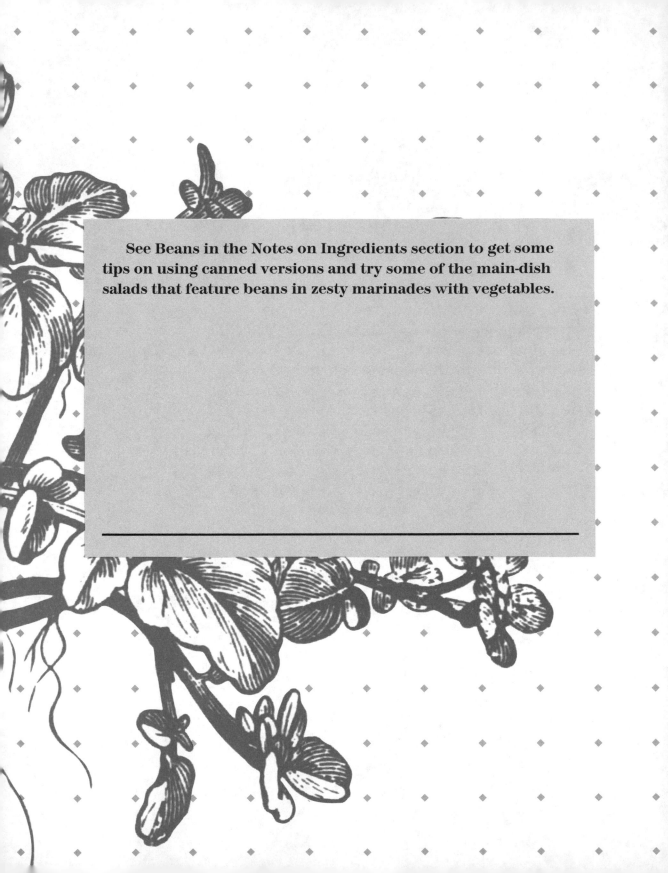

See Beans in the Notes on Ingredients section to get some tips on using canned versions and try some of the main-dish salads that feature beans in zesty marinades with vegetables.

Quick CHEESE AND BEAN QUESADILLAS

When quesadillas are filled only with cheese, they are too rich for me. Adding beans, olives, and scallions improves the texture and flavor of the filling. The recipe can be easily multiplied (make sure you have 2 baking sheets) and makes wonderful informal party food.

2 cups grated Monterey Jack cheese with jalapeño peppers

1 cup cooked kidney beans, rinsed and drained if canned

1 scallion, very thinly sliced

10 pitted black olives (California-style), thinly sliced

1 tablespoon finely chopped cilantro

4 8-inch flour (wheat) tortillas

Serves 2

1 Preheat the oven to 375 degrees.

2 In a large bowl, combine the cheese, beans, scallion, olives, and cilantro.

3 Place 2 tortillas side by side on a baking sheet. Divide the mixture and spread onto each tortilla, leaving a 1-inch border. Press the filling down with your fingers. Cover with the remaining 2 tortillas and press down again.

4 Bake 10 minutes, or until the cheese is thoroughly melted. Cut each quesadilla into 4 wedges before serving.

Quick VEGETABLE AND BLACK BEAN BURRITOS

Mixing vegetables with beans makes these delectable burritos significantly lighter than traditional bean burritos, while the inclusion of orange in this spicy filling adds a dazzling touch. I have come to enjoy making burritos a lot more since some friends showed me this clever method of steaming wheat tortillas. It's easy and quick, and it makes the tortillas very tender. Lay out the fillings for the burritos and let each person make his or her own, steaming the tortillas as needed.

1 tablespoon vegetable oil

1 medium onion, finely diced

1 large red or green bell pepper, cored and finely diced

1 16-ounce can black beans, rinsed and drained

1¼ cups frozen corn kernels, thawed

5 orange sections, each cut into ½-inch dice

1¼ cups salsa, medium or hot

....

8 wheat (flour) tortillas (about 8 inches in diameter)

1½ cups grated sharp Cheddar cheese

Sour cream

Serves 4 (8 burritos)

1 Heat the oil in a large skillet over medium heat. Add the onion and pepper and sauté until very tender, about 10 minutes.

2 Add the black beans, corn, and oranges and cook 2 minutes, or until heated through. Stir in the salsa, then remove the pan from the heat.

3 Fill a pot that is at least 8 inches in diameter with about 2 inches of water. Cover the pot with a piece of foil, making it tight and secure. With a knife tip, poke holes all over the top of the foil. Bring the water to a boil, then place a tortilla on the foil. Steam it for about 1 minute, flip it over, and steam it on the other side for about 30 seconds, or just until hot. Repeat with the remaining tortillas as needed.

4 To serve, place a tortilla on a large plate. Spoon an eighth of the bean mixture along the center of the tortilla, then top with some cheese and a bit of sour cream. Roll, eat, and enjoy.

BAKED VEGETABLES WITH GARLIC, WHITE BEANS, AND OLIVES

This *Mediterranean-style casserole, layered with cheese, needs only some crusty bread to accompany it and to sop up any garlicky juices left on your plate.*

1 large bunch broccoli, cut into small florets

3 medium-large boiling potatoes, peeled and cut into 1-inch chunks

1 28-ounce can tomatoes, finely chopped and well drained

1 15-ounce can cannellini (white beans), rinsed and drained

½ cup pitted black olives, halved (any style; see note, page xx)

2½ tablespoons olive oil

4 garlic cloves, minced

¼ teaspoon crushed red pepper flakes

Salt

1¼ cups (4 ounces) grated Muenster cheese

Serves 3 to 4

1 Bring a 3-quart saucepan of water to a boil. Blanch the broccoli for 2 minutes, or until tender yet still crunchy. Remove with a slotted spoon, then plunge into a bowl of cold water to stop the cooking. Drain well and pat dry. Place in a large bowl.

2 Drop the potatoes into the boiling water and cook until tender, about 7 minutes. Drain well and add to the broccoli.

3 Stir in the tomatoes, cannellini, and olives. Combine the olive oil, garlic, and red pepper flakes. Pour over the vegetables and toss gently to coat. Season with salt to taste.

4 Preheat the oven to 400 degrees.

5 Spread half the vegetable mixture in a shallow casserole, such as a 12 × 7 × 2-inch Pyrex dish. Sprinkle on half the Muenster cheese. Spoon on the remaining vegetables, then top with the remaining cheese. Cover the dish with foil.

6 Bake 30 minutes, or until hot and bubbly. Remove the foil and bake 5 additional minutes for a golden crust.

CORN PANCAKES TOPPED WITH BLACK BEANS

R uth Bronz, chef at the Bronze Dog Cafe in Great Barrington, Massachusetts, serves a fabulous combination of buttery corn pancakes topped with a mound of creamy black beans. After indulging in that great dish, I rushed home and created this version.

THE BLACK BEANS

1 tablespoon olive oil

1 garlic clove, pressed or minced

½ teaspoon ground cumin

2 16-ounce cans black beans, rinsed and drained

A few dashes of Tabasco sauce, or to taste

¾ cup water

CORN PANCAKES

1½ cups unbleached flour

2 tablespoons sugar

2 teaspoons baking powder

1 teaspoon salt

3 eggs

1¼ cups low-fat milk

2 tablespoons butter, melted

2 cups frozen corn kernels, thawed

Oil for greasing

Sour cream

Serves 4 (12 4-inch pancakes)

1 Heat the oil in a medium-size saucepan over medium heat. Add the garlic and cumin and sauté 1 minute. Stir in the black beans, Tabasco, and water and bring to a boil. Reduce the heat to a lively simmer and cook the mixture 5 minutes. Remove from the heat and let cool slightly.

2 Pour the contents of the pot into a food processor or blender and process until the beans are creamy yet still chunky. Scrape the mixture back into the saucepan and keep warm over low heat.

3 To make the pancakes, combine the flour, sugar, baking powder, and salt in a large bowl and mix well.

4 In a blender or food processor, thoroughly blend the eggs, milk, and melted butter. Add the corn and process a few seconds until almost puréed. You want to retain some chunks. Pour this mixture into the flour and stir just until blended. Do not overmix.

5 Lightly coat a griddle or large skillet with some oil and heat over medium heat until a drop of water dances when flicked on the pan.

6 Drop tablespoons of batter onto the griddle to make 4-inch pancakes. Cook until golden brown on each side; to make sure they are cooked through, make a slit in the center and peek at them. The batter should yield about 12 pancakes.

7 Meanwhile, check the consistency of the black beans; they should be like very soft mashed potatoes. If they are too thick, stir in a little water; if they are too soupy, cook them a little more.

8 On each plate, arrange 3 pancakes slightly overlapping in the center. Spoon some of the black beans onto the center and garnish with a small spoonful of sour cream.

Note: If you have leftover batter, cover and refrigerate; it will keep for 48 hours.

BAKED TOFU SZECHUAN STYLE

Quick

I came across this idea of baking marinated tofu at a health food supermarket. It is so easy and so flavorful that it has now become my favorite way to prepare tofu. Serve it with a grain dish such as couscous, rice, or bulghur pilaf.

THE MARINADE

2 tablespoons tamari soy sauce

1 tablespoon Oriental sesame oil

1 tablespoon vegetable oil

½ teaspoon minced fresh ginger

....

1 pound extra-firm tofu, cut into ¾-inch cubes and patted very dry

THE SAUCE

½ to 1 teaspoon chili paste with garlic

1 tablespoon tahini or natural-style peanut butter

2 tablespoons dry sherry, rice wine, or vermouth

Serves 3

1 In a medium-size bowl, combine the marinade ingredients. Gently stir in the tofu and coat well. Let marinate for 30 minutes, or up to 8 hours. Cover and chill if longer than 30 minutes.

2 Preheat the oven to 450 degrees.

3 Pour the tofu and its marinade into a shallow baking dish in one layer. Bake for 15 minutes, tossing once with a spatula.

4 Combine the sauce ingredients and pour over the tofu. Toss to coat evenly. Return to the oven and bake 10 more minutes, or until golden brown. Let sit 10 minutes before serving; it should be served warm, not piping hot.

Quick STIR-FRIED BROCCOLI AND TOFU IN PEANUT SAUCE

This spicy peanut sauce laced with ginger and garlic is the perfect foil for mild tofu. Cook 1 cup of rice before you begin stir-frying and keep it warm on the back burner.

THE SAUCE

¼ cup natural-style peanut butter

3 tablespoons tamari soy sauce

3 tablespoons Chinese rice wine or sherry

2 tablespoons water

1 tablespoon Oriental sesame oil

....

2 tablespoons vegetable oil

1 pound extra-firm tofu, cut into ½-inch cubes and patted very dry

3 garlic cloves, minced

1 teaspoon minced fresh ginger

¼ teaspoon crushed red pepper flakes

1 bunch broccoli, stalks peeled and cut into small pieces (about 5 cups)

¼ cup water

Hot cooked rice

Serves 4

1 Combine the peanut butter, tamari, and rice wine or sherry in a small bowl or large measuring cup and beat with a fork until smooth. Stir in the water and sesame oil, then set aside.

2 Heat 1 tablespoon of the vegetable oil in a large skillet or wok over medium-high heat until it is very hot but not smoking. Make sure the tofu is very dry, then drop it in the pan. Stir-fry until golden all over, about 10 minutes. Remove to a platter.

3 Add the remaining tablespoon of oil to the pan. Stir in the garlic, ginger, and crushed pepper flakes. Cook 2 minutes, stirring constantly. Do not let the garlic brown.

4 Add the broccoli, toss, then pour in the ¼ cup water. Cover the pan and cook the broccoli about 5 minutes, or until bright green and slightly crunchy. Remove the cover occasionally to toss the broccoli.

5 Return the tofu to the pan and toss. Pour on the peanut sauce and stir-fry 1 minute. Serve on rice.

Quick BARBECUED TOFU WITH PEPPERS AND ONIONS

The surprise ingredient in this barbecue sauce is a small amount of peanut butter, which helps the sauce adhere to the tofu and make it crispy. This treatment also works well on the grill. Cook the tofu and vegetables on skewers, rotating occasionally until evenly browned.

1 pound extra-firm tofu, cut into ¾-inch cubes and patted very dry

1 green pepper, cored and cut into 1-inch squares

2 small onions, quartered vertically, sections separated into halves

2 tablespoons tamari soy sauce

1 tablespoon vegetable oil

THE SAUCE

1 tablespoon natural-style peanut butter

1 teaspoon vegetable oil

2½ tablespoons ketchup

1 teaspoon mustard

2 teaspoons apple cider vinegar

2 garlic cloves, pressed

2 teaspoons chili powder

1 teaspoon molasses

A few dashes of Tabasco sauce

Generous seasoning of freshly ground pepper

Serves 3

1 Place the tofu in a large bowl with the pepper and onions.

2 Combine the tamari and oil and pour over the vegetables. With a rubber spatula, toss gently to coat. Let marinate for at least 30 minutes, or up to 4 hours.

3 Mix together all the ingredients for the sauce. Let sit at least 30 minutes to allow the flavors to meld.

4 Preheat the oven to 450 degrees.

5 Scrape the tofu and vegetables into a 9 × 13-inch baking dish, or similar large, shallow baking dish, ample enough for everything to rest in one layer. Bake for 15 minutes, tossing once with a spatula.

6 Remove the baking dish from the oven. Spoon on the sauce and gently toss to coat evenly. Return to the oven and bake 15 more minutes, or until lightly browned. Let sit 10 minutes so it can be served warm, not hot.

Quick TOFU HOISIN WITH BROCCOLI, RED PEPPER, AND WALNUTS

The garlic and hot pep-
per flakes are a nice foil for the sweetness of
the hoisin sauce. To organize yourself, cook 1½
cups rice before you begin stir-frying and keep
it warm on the back burner; the stir-frying will
take only a few minutes.

THE SAUCE

⅓ cup hoisin sauce

2 tablespoons Chinese rice
wine or dry sherry

1 tablespoon Oriental
sesame oil

1 tablespoon tamari soy
sauce

....

2 tablespoons vegetable oil

1 pound extra-firm tofu,
sliced, patted very dry,
then cut into 2 × ½-inch
logs

6 garlic cloves, minced

⅛ teaspoon crushed red
pepper flakes

1 red bell pepper, cut into
3 × ½-inch strips

1 bunch broccoli, cut into
small florets, stalks peeled
and sliced (about 5 cups)

½ cup walnut halves

⅓ cup water

Serves 3 to 4

1 Combine all the sauce ingredients in a small bowl and set aside.

2 Heat the oil in a wok or large skillet over high heat until it is hot but not smoking. Make sure the tofu is patted very dry to prevent sticking. Add the tofu and stir-fry until lightly golden all over. Remove to a platter and reduce the heat to medium-high.

3 If there is no oil left in the pan, add a teaspoon or so. Add the garlic and crushed pepper flakes and cook 1 minute. Stir in the red bell pepper, broccoli, and walnuts and toss to coat with the garlic. Pour in the water, toss, then cover the pan. Cook 5 minutes, or until the vegetables are tender yet still crunchy.

4 Stir in the tofu, then pour on the sauce mixture. Stir-fry 1 minute, or until the sauce coats everything and is thickened. Serve on rice.

Quick TEMPEH FAJITAS WITH CUCUMBER SALSA

Marinated tempeh and peppers are "roasted" to fill these fajitas, making them a very nutritious choice for either lunch or supper.

THE MARINADE

3 tablespoons tamari soy sauce

Juice of ½ lime

1 teaspoon brown sugar

2 tablespoons vegetable oil

3 garlic cloves, minced

¼ teaspoon crushed red pepper flakes

THE FILLING

8 ounces tempeh, cut into 3 × ½-inch strips

1 yellow bell pepper, cut into ½-inch strips

1 red bell pepper, cut into ½-inch strips

1 green bell pepper, cut into ½-inch strips

1 medium red onion, halved vertically and thinly sliced

CUCUMBER SALSA

⅔ cup low-fat yogurt

½ small cucumber, peeled, seeded, and finely diced (about ⅓ cup)

1 Combine the marinade ingredients in a large bowl. Stir in the tempeh, bell peppers, and onion. Marinate for at least 30 minutes, or up to 2 hours.

2 In a small bowl, combine the salsa ingredients. Cover and chill until ready to use.

3 Preheat the oven to 450 degrees.

4 Sprinkle a little water on each tortilla and rub it around the tortilla with your fingers. Stack the tortillas, then wrap the bundle in foil. Set aside.

5 Spread the marinated tempeh and vegetables on a baking sheet in one layer. Bake 15 minutes, or until the vegetables are tender and the tempeh begins to brown. Do not toss while cooking.

6 Place the tortilla packet in the oven for about 7 minutes. This will heat the tortillas with a little "steam" to soften them.

7 To serve, place a tortilla on each plate. Spoon some of the tempeh mixture along the center, cover with a little cucumber salsa, then fold and roll to enclose the filling.

¼ teaspoon ground cumin

1 tablespoon minced fresh parsley

....

8 8-inch flour tortillas

Serves 4

BLACK BEAN CAKES WITH ORANGE BASIL SALSA

Tomatoes and oranges together in salsa make a great match both for flavor and dynamic color. Serve these hearty bean cakes with a rice pilaf sprinkled with scallions.

SALSA

2 navel oranges, sections separated and cut into small dice

1 large tomato, cored, sliced, and finely diced

1 scallion, very thinly sliced

1 tablespoon minced fresh basil

1 garlic clove, minced

1 tablespoon lime juice

2 teaspoons olive oil

1 small jalapeño pepper, seeded and minced (wear gloves), or ¼ teaspoon crushed red pepper flakes

Salt

THE BEAN CAKES

4 cups cooked black beans, rinsed and drained if canned

2 eggs

½ cup bread crumbs

1 tablespoon olive oil, plus oil for greasing pan

1 Combine all the salsa ingredients in a bowl. Let sit at least 1 hour, or up to 8 hours, before using.

2 Place 3 cups of the black beans in a large bowl. Process the remaining 1 cup of beans with the eggs until smooth. Stir this mixture into the whole beans along with the bread crumbs.

3 Heat the oil in a medium skillet over medium heat. Add the onion, garlic, and celery and sauté until very tender and beginning to brown, about 10 minutes. Sprinkle on the cumin and cook 1 more minute.

4 Scrape the vegetables into the bean mixture and add the salt and pepper. Stir to mix well.

5 Preheat the oven to 375 degrees. Lightly oil a baking sheet.

6 Using a ⅓ cup measuring cup, scoop up 12 portions of the bean mixture and place on the baking sheet. With a knife or your hands, flatten into patty shapes. Bake 10 minutes, flip with a spatula, and bake 10 more minutes. Serve the bean cakes with a spoonful of salsa on each.

 Note: The dish may be prepared in advance through step 4. Cover and refrigerate for up to 8 hours.

1 medium onion, very finely diced

2 garlic cloves, minced

1 celery rib, very thinly sliced

1 teaspoon ground cumin

¼ teaspoon salt

Liberal seasoning of freshly ground pepper

Serves 4 to 6

Quick SAVORY WHITE BEANS WITH RED ONION AND FRESH HERBS

I *love white beans, especially cannellini and Great Northern. This easy method of serving them as a main course accentuates their buttery flavor. I serve this dish with sautéed spinach, which adds just the right color and texture.*

1½ tablespoons olive oil

2 celery ribs, thinly sliced

1 medium red onion, quartered and cut into ¼-inch slices

1½ teaspoons red wine vinegar

1 tomato, cored, seeded, and finely diced

6 fresh sage leaves, finely chopped, or ¼ teaspoon powdered dried

2 sprigs fresh thyme, finely chopped, or ½ teaspoon dried

¼ cup chopped fresh parsley

4 cups freshly cooked white beans, such as cannellini or Great Northern, or 2 15-ounce cans white beans, rinsed thoroughly and drained

Salt

Generous seasoning of freshly ground pepper

Serves 4

1 Heat the oil in a large skillet over medium heat. Add the celery and sauté 5 minutes, stirring often.

2 Add the onion and cook 2 minutes. Pour the vinegar over the vegetables to set the color of the red onion; toss to coat well. Sauté about 5 minutes, or until the onion is tender.

3 Stir in the tomato and cook 2 minutes. Mix in all the remaining ingredients and cook about 5 more minutes, or until piping hot. If the mixture is dry, sprinkle on a few teaspoons of water and toss to blend. The beans should be moist and juicy, not dry.

Quick CORN AND BEAN TOSTADAS

▼▼▼▼▼▼▼▼▼▼

Mexicans cleverly use
nuts in their main-course cooking, especially as
thickening agents. Here, walnuts add a delightful crunch to this flavorful topping. A light salad
is all you need to accompany this dish.

1½ tablespoons vegetable oil

4 8-inch flour (wheat) tortillas

1 15-ounce can kidney beans, rinsed and well drained

1 cup frozen corn kernels, thawed

½ cup sliced black olives

¼ cup finely chopped cilantro

⅓ cup finely chopped walnuts (not ground)

½ cup mild or medium salsa

2 cups (6 ounces) grated Monterey Jack cheese with jalapeño peppers

Serves 2 to 3

1 Preheat the broiler.

2 With a vegetable brush, lightly coat 2 tortillas on both sides with some of the vegetable oil. Place on a baking sheet and broil until lightly golden on one side. Flip over and broil again until golden. Repeat with the remaining tortillas. Let cool on a rack. (You can prepare the tortillas up to 24 hours in advance; keep them covered in the refrigerator.)

3 Preheat the oven to 375 degrees.

4 In a large bowl, combine the kidney beans, corn, olives, cilantro, walnuts, and salsa.

5 Using two baking sheets or cooking just 2 tortillas at a time, divide the bean mixture and spread on each tortilla. Sprinkle on the cheese.

6 Bake 7 to 10 minutes, or until hot and bubbly. Slice in half before serving.

VEGETABLE DAL

Dal is an Indian purée made of lentils or split peas and spices. Here it is prepared like a stew with vegetables (called sambaar) and served on rice. If you have never eaten dal, you're in for a taste awakening. The blending of flavors is dazzling. Cook about 1 ½ cups rice (preferably basmati rice) to serve with this sambaar, and don't hesitate to make the sambaar up to 24 hours in advance; its flavor will be heightened as a result of sitting.

1 cup yellow split peas

4 cups water

1 teaspoon salt

....

2 tablespoons vegetable oil

2 medium onions, finely diced

2 garlic cloves, minced

½ teaspoon turmeric

1 teaspoon ground coriander

1 teaspoon ground cumin

¼ teaspoon cayenne

1 tomato, cored, seeded, and finely diced

1 cup water

2 medium potatoes, peeled and cut into ½-inch dice

8 ounces fresh spinach, stems discarded and leaves chopped into small pieces (about 8 cups loosely packed)

1 teaspoon lemon juice

1 Rinse the split peas in a sieve under cold running water. Pick out and discard any stones or foreign particles. Place the split peas in a 3-quart saucepan along with the water and salt. Bring to a boil, then reduce the heat to a simmer. Cook, stirring occasionally, for 45 minutes. Skim off and discard any foam that rises to the surface.

2 Meanwhile, heat the vegetable oil in a large skillet over medium-high heat. Add the onions and garlic and sauté until they begin to turn brown, about 15 minutes. Stir often. Mix in all the spices and cook 2 more minutes. Add the tomato and cook 2 minutes.

3 Pour in the cup of water and bring to a boil. Stir in the potatoes, cover the pan, and reduce the heat to a simmer. Cook until the potatoes are just about tender, about 10 minutes.

4 When the split peas are very soft and almost a purée, stir vigorously to make them smoother. Carefully stir in the contents of the skillet along with the spinach and lemon juice. Cook, stirring frequently to prevent sticking, 10 to 15 more

1 tablespoon finely chopped cilantro

2 tablespoons unsalted butter

Serves 4 to 6

minutes, or until the dal is the consistency of a thick stew and the vegetables are tender. (If too thick, add a little water.) Stir in the cilantro and butter and cook 2 more minutes. Serve on rice.

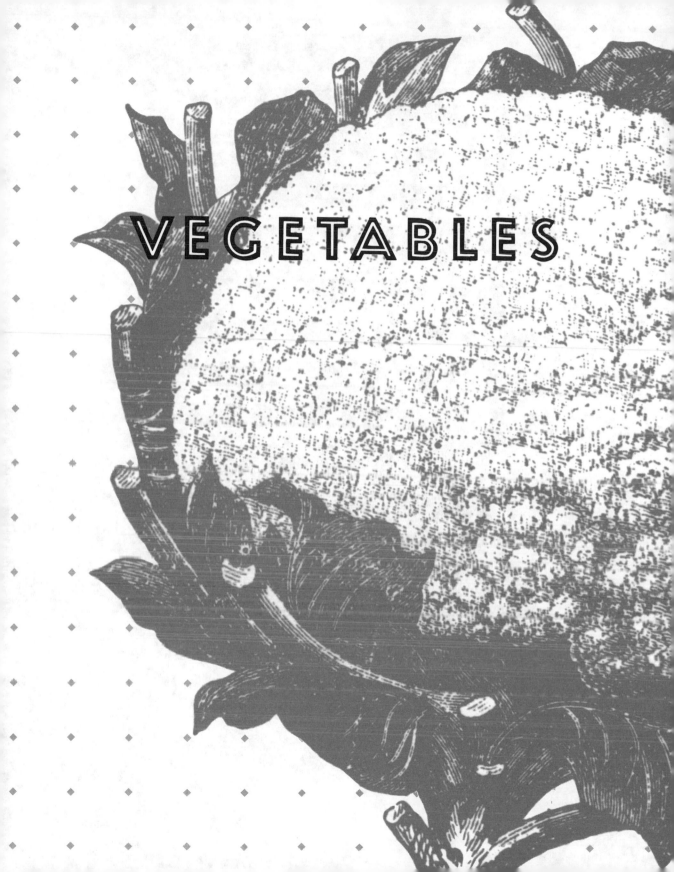

VEGETABLES

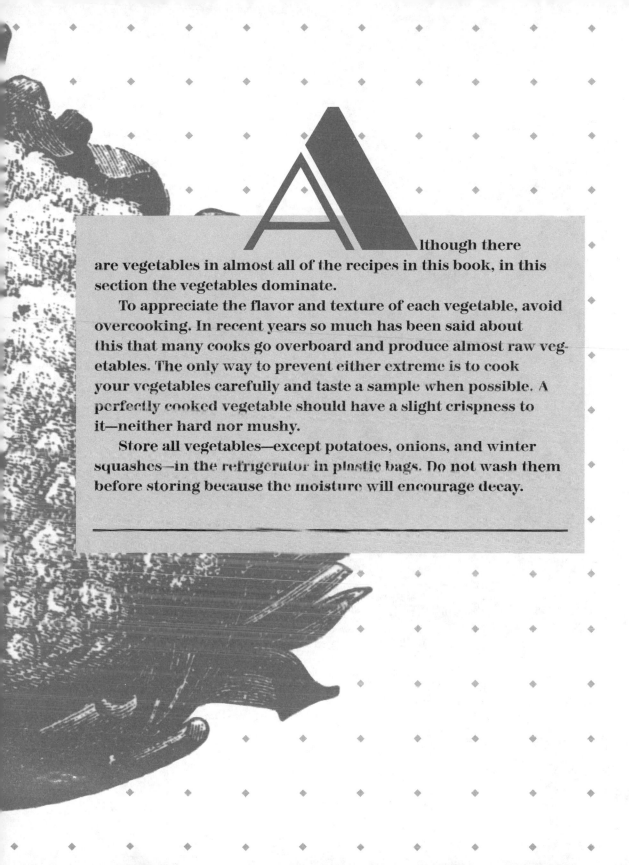

Although there are vegetables in almost all of the recipes in this book, in this section the vegetables dominate.

To appreciate the flavor and texture of each vegetable, avoid overcooking. In recent years so much has been said about this that many cooks go overboard and produce almost raw vegetables. The only way to prevent either extreme is to cook your vegetables carefully and taste a sample when possible. A perfectly cooked vegetable should have a slight crispness to it—neither hard nor mushy.

Store all vegetables—except potatoes, onions, and winter squashes—in the refrigerator in plastic bags. Do not wash them before storing because the moisture will encourage decay.

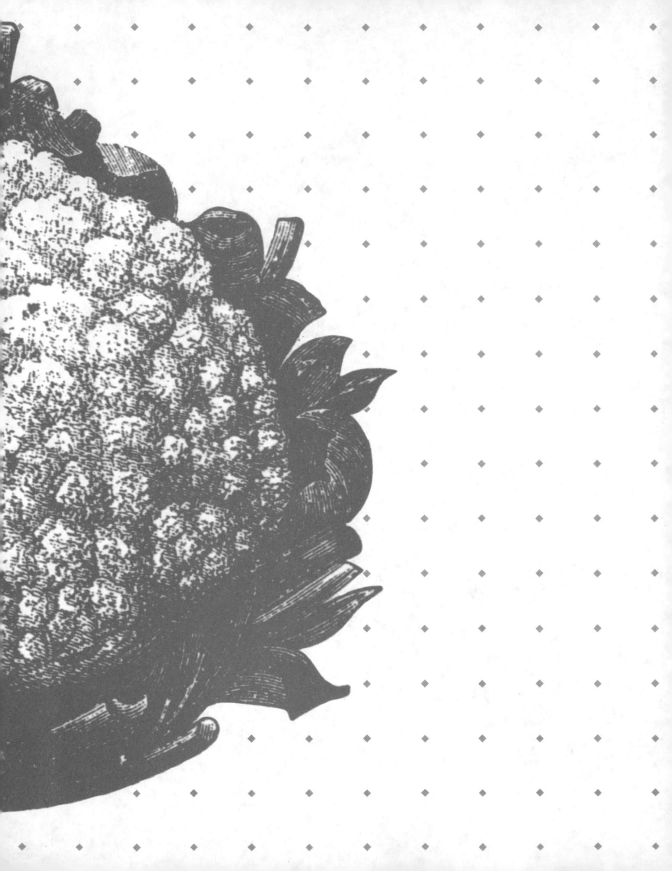

BAKED GARLICKY BUTTERNUT SQUASH

Here is a variation of a recipe that the late Laurie Colwin wrote in Gourmet. This crusty, garlic-scented dish needs just a salad to make it a completely satisfying and delicious meal, although a close friend of mine says it is absolutely spellbinding served on a golden bed of polenta.

1 large (3½ pounds) butternut squash, peeled and cut into 1-inch dice

⅓ cup fruity olive oil

2 garlic cloves, minced

2 tablespoons minced fresh parsley

Salt to taste

Liberal seasoning of freshly ground pepper

¼ cup grated Parmesan cheese

Serves 4

1 Preheat the oven to 400 degrees.

2 In a large bowl, toss together the squash, olive oil, garlic, parsley, salt, and pepper.

3 Spoon the vegetables into a 12 × 7 × 2-inch Pyrex dish or other shallow 2½-quart baking dish. Sprinkle on the Parmesan cheese. Bake for 1 hour, or until the squash is tender, not mushy.

CRUSTLESS SPINACH AND MUSHROOM PIE

This easy pie goes well with a potato side dish. It's just as delicious reheated, so look forward to a tasty lunch of leftovers.

2 10-ounce packages fresh spinach, washed and chopped, or 2 10-ounce packages frozen chopped spinach, thawed and squeezed dry

½ tablespoon unsalted butter

¼ cup bread crumbs

1 tablespoon olive oil

12 ounces (4½ cups) sliced mushrooms

2 scallions, thinly sliced

3 eggs

¾ cup low-fat milk

1 cup grated extra-sharp Cheddar cheese

⅛ teaspoon grated nutmeg

½ teaspoon salt

Freshly ground pepper

Serves 4

1 Prepare either the fresh or defrosted spinach as directed and set aside.

2 Preheat the oven to 375 degrees. With the butter, coat the inside of a 9-inch pie plate, then sprinkle with bread crumbs, rotating the plate to cover the sides. Let the extra crumbs fall to the bottom; this will form the crust.

3 In a large skillet, heat the olive oil over medium-high heat. Add the mushrooms and sauté until brown and the juices have evaporated, about 10 minutes. If you are using fresh spinach, add it with just the water that clings to it. Cover the pan. Cook until the spinach just wilts, about 5 minutes. If you are using frozen spinach, stir it into the mushrooms.

4 Stir in the scallions, then remove the pan from the heat and let cool.

5 In a large bowl, beat the eggs. Beat in the milk, all but 2 tablespoons of the Cheddar cheese, the nutmeg, salt, and pepper. Stir in the cooled spinach mixture.

6 Scrape everything into the prepared pie plate. Sprinkle the remaining Cheddar cheese evenly over the top.

7 Bake 30 minutes, or until a knife inserted in the center of the pie comes out clean. Cool for a few minutes before serving; cut into wedges.

❧ *Note:* May be prepared up to 8 hours in advance through step 5 and refrigerated. Bring to room temperature before baking.

BROCCOLI AND RED PEPPER PIE

This colorful pie with a bread crumb "crust" has an added boost of protein from the chickpeas sprinkled throughout. For a pleasing accompaniment, try serving it with buttered egg noodles.

1 tablespoon olive oil

2 garlic cloves, minced

2 medium onions, finely diced

⅛ teaspoon crushed red pepper flakes

5 cups tiny broccoli florets (from 1 large bunch)

1 large red bell pepper, cored and diced

½ cup cooked, rinsed chickpeas (see note)

....

1 tablespoon unsalted butter, softened

¼ cup plus 1 tablespoon bread crumbs

....

3 eggs

½ cup milk

¼ cup grated Parmesan cheese

¼ teaspoon dried oregano

1 Heat the oil in a large skillet over medium-high heat. Add the garlic, onions, and red pepper flakes and sauté for 10 minutes.

2 Stir in the broccoli, crushed red pepper flakes, and chickpeas. Pour on 2 tablespoons of water, cover the pan, and cook for about 7 minutes, or until the broccoli is tender yet still bright green. Remove the cover and cook away any remaining liquid. Place the mixture in a bowl and let cool.

3 Preheat the oven to 375 degrees.

4 To make the "crust," butter a 9-inch pie plate with ½ tablespoon of the soft butter. Sprinkle ¼ cup of bread crumbs on the bottom of the pie plate. Rotate to cover the bottom and sides of the plate with the crumbs.

5 In a large bowl, beat the eggs. Beat in the milk, Parmesan cheese, oregano, salt, and pepper. Stir in the vegetable mixture. Spoon half the mixture into the pie plate. Sprinkle on the Muenster cheese. Spoon on the remaining mixture, then sprinkle the remaining tablespoon of bread crumbs over the top. Dot with the remaining ½ tablespoon butter.

¼ teaspoon salt

Liberal seasoning of
freshly ground pepper

1 cup (3 ounces) grated
Muenster cheese

Serves 3 to 4

6 Bake 30 to 35 minutes, or until a knife inserted
in the center of the pie comes out clean. Let sit
5 minutes before serving.

 Note: Leftover chickpeas can be marinated in
an herb vinaigrette and served in a salad at
another time.

Quick VEGETABLE TIAN

A tian is a Provençal shallow earthenware casserole, which gives this vegetable dish its name. Other shallow baking dishes can do a similar job of slowly baking a vegetable concoction in olive oil and herbs.

Try to make this dish as is without improvisation because the balance of juicy and dry vegetables provides just the right amount of moisture to ensure even cooking. The heavenly crumb topping made of fresh bread crumbs gives this tian added depth, so be sure to include it. To add to the meal, try a side dish of egg noodles. My husband and I are so enamored of this tian that the two of us can polish off the whole thing with just a bit of French bread as an accompaniment.

2 slices good-quality white bread

1 tablespoon plus ¼ cup olive oil

1 garlic clove, minced

1 pound green beans, tips removed

12 ounces mushrooms, halved or quartered, depending on size

1 red bell pepper, cut into 2-inch chunks

1 tomato, seeded and finely diced

1 large red onion, cut into eighths

½ teaspoon dried basil

½ teaspoon dried oregano

1 teaspoon dried dill weed

Generous seasoning of freshly ground pepper

Serves 4

1 Preheat the oven to 375 degrees.

2 Tear the bread into pieces. Place them in a blender or food processor and make bread crumbs.

3 Heat 1 tablespoon olive oil in a small skillet over medium heat. Add the garlic and sauté 1 minute. Stir in the crumbs and toss to coat thoroughly with the oil. Cook, stirring frequently, until the crumbs begin to turn golden and crisp, about 5 minutes. Remove from the heat.

4 In a large bowl, combine all the remaining ingredients, including the remaining ¼ cup olive oil. Toss well. Scrape the mixture into a shallow 2½-quart baking dish and smooth over the top. Sprinkle on the bread crumbs and press them down evenly. Bake 1 hour, or until the vegetables are very tender.

TWICE-BAKED POTATOES STUFFED WITH CHEESE AND SALSA

Even though these potatoes must be cooked an hour before being stuffed, I think of them as very quick to prepare because they take only 10 minutes of my time. This low-fat, high-protein version of stuffed potatoes needs just a salad to complete the meal.

2 large baking potatoes, scrubbed

½ cup low-fat cottage cheese

1 tablespoon low-fat milk

½ cup grated part-skim mozzarella cheese

3 tablespoons mild, medium, or hot salsa

2 tablespoons minced fresh parsley

Serves 2

1 Preheat the oven to 400 degrees.

2 Poke the potatoes a few times with the tip of a knife. Place them directly on the rack in the oven and bake until tender when pierced through the center, about 1 hour.

3 Meanwhile, blend the cottage cheese and milk together in a blender or food processor until perfectly smooth. Scrape into a bowl and stir in the mozzarella, salsa, and parsley.

4 When the potatoes are done, slice them in half lengthwise. Scoop the flesh into a medium-size bowl. Mash it with a fork, then stir in the cheese mixture. Fill each potato shell with some filling.

5 Place the stuffed potatoes on a baking sheet. Bake 20 minutes, or until brown on top.

MUSHROOM ENCHILADAS

Cottage cheese enhances the tasty filling in these enchiladas. Because they are so satisfying, a salad is all you need to balance the meal.

1 tablespoon olive oil

2 garlic cloves, minced

1 pound mushrooms, thinly sliced (about 6 cups)

½ teaspoon dried oregano

1 16-ounce can pinto beans, rinsed and well drained

1 cup low-fat small curd cottage cheese

½ cup finely chopped fresh parsley

2 cups mild or medium salsa

8 8-inch flour (wheat) tortillas

1 cup grated sharp Cheddar cheese

Serves 4 to 6

1 Heat the oil in a large skillet over medium-high heat. Add the garlic and cook 1 minute. Do not burn it. Stir in the mushrooms and cook until the juices are released and then evaporate, about 10 minutes. The mushrooms should begin to stick to the pan.

2 Add the oregano and pinto beans and cook 1 minute. Remove the pan from the heat and let the mixture cool.

3 Preheat the oven to 375 degrees.

4 Stir the cottage cheese and parsley into the bean mixture. Place the pan in front of you to begin rolling the enchiladas. Place the salsa in a bowl in front of you, along with the tortillas and a pastry brush.

5 Spread a thin layer of salsa in a 9 × 13-inch baking dish. Lay a tortilla on a plate, then brush both sides of the tortilla with a little bit of salsa. This will moisten the tortillas and prevent them from breaking. Divide the mushroom mixture into 8 portions and place 1 portion along the bottom of a tortilla. Roll tightly. Place the enchilada seam side down in the baking dish. Repeat with the remaining tortillas.

6 Spoon the remaining salsa all over the enchiladas. Neatly place the Cheddar cheese along each enchilada. Cover the baking dish tightly with foil.

7 Bake 30 minutes, then remove the foil and bake 5 more minutes. The enchiladas should be piping hot, but be careful not to dry them out through overcooking.

~ *Note:* The enchiladas can be prepared up to 8 hours in advance through step 6. Bring to room temperature before baking.

Quick MIXED PEPPER QUESADILLAS

▼▼▼▼▼▼▼▼▼▼▼▼

The filling in these quesadillas is scrumptious. They make a great choice for lunch or dinner.

1 tablespoon olive oil

1 red bell pepper, cored and cut into very thin strips

1 yellow bell pepper, cored and cut into very thin strips

1 green bell pepper, cored and cut into very thin strips

1 tomato, cored, seeded, and finely diced

8 pitted black olives, thinly sliced

1 teaspoon red wine vinegar

1 teaspoon oregano

Salt

Generous seasoning of freshly ground pepper

. . . .

4 8-inch flour (wheat) tortillas

1¼ cups grated Monterey Jack cheese with jalapeño peppers

Serves 2 to 3

1 Heat the oil in a large skillet over medium-high heat. Add the peppers and sauté, tossing often, for 10 minutes, or until the peppers are tender.

2 Stir in the tomato, olives, vinegar, oregano, salt, and pepper and cook until the peppers are very soft, about 10 more minutes. Remove from the heat and let the mixture cool.

3 Preheat the oven to 375 degrees.

4 Place 2 of the tortillas on a baking sheet. Sprinkle a quarter of the cheese on each tortilla, leaving a 1-inch border. Spread half the pepper mixture on each tortilla, then sprinkle on the remaining cheese. Top with the remaining tortillas, gently pressing down to make the filling adhere.

5 Bake 10 minutes, or until the cheese is thoroughly melted. Cut each quesadilla into 4 wedges before serving.

Quick LEEK FRITTATA

It's unfortunate that leeks aren't as popular in the United States as they are in Europe because their sweet delicate flavor is incomparable. Serve this delicious frittata with home fries and toasted peasant-style bread for a great trio.

3 large leeks

1 tablespoon unsalted butter

6 eggs

¼ cup low-fat milk

2 tablespoons grated Parmesan cheese

¼ teaspoon salt

Freshly ground pepper

Serves 3 to 4

1 Cut the roots off the leeks. Cut off all but about 3 inches of the dark green part and discard. Make a vertical cut down the length of the leeks almost through to the back. Wash the leeks very thoroughly under cold running water, separating the leaves to reveal any hidden dirt. Pat the leeks dry, then thinly slice them, discarding any tough green part if necessary. (You should have about 3½ cups.)

2 Preheat the oven to 350 degrees. Butter a 9-inch pie plate and set aside.

3 Melt the tablespoon of butter in a large skillet over medium heat. Add the leeks and sauté, stirring often, until tender, about 10 minutes. Set aside to cool.

4 Beat the eggs in a large bowl. Beat in the milk, cheese, salt, and pepper, then stir in the leeks. Pour this mixture into the pie plate.

5 Bake 20 to 25 minutes, or just until a knife inserted in the center comes out clean. Do not overcook. Serve immediately.

Quick SUMMER FRITTATA

This frittata is light on eggs and chock-full of vegetables—a good choice when you have small amounts of several vegetables on hand. Plan ahead so you can serve it warm, not hot; the texture and flavor will be improved.

1 tablespoon olive oil

1 small zucchini, finely diced

1 small yellow squash, finely diced

1 red bell pepper, finely diced

1 tomato, cored, seeded, and finely diced

4 scallions, very thinly sliced

¼ cup shredded fresh basil, or ½ teaspoon dried

Butter for greasing

4 eggs

¼ teaspoon salt

1 cup grated Monterey Jack cheese with jalapeño peppers

Serves 4 generously

1 Heat the oil in a large skillet over medium-high heat. Add the zucchini, yellow squash, and red pepper and sauté until the vegetables begin to get tender, about 7 minutes.

2 Add the tomato and continue to cook the mixture, tossing often, until the vegetables are tender and the mixture begins to stick to the pan. Raise the heat to evaporate any excess juices. Remove from the heat, then stir in the scallions and basil. Let the mixture cool.

3 Preheat the oven to 350 degrees. Butter a 9-inch pie plate.

4 Beat the eggs and salt in a large bowl. Stir in the cheese and vegetable mixture and pour into the pie plate.

5 Bake 25 to 28 minutes, or until a knife inserted in the center of the frittata comes out dry. Cool the frittata on a rack and serve it warm, not hot.

Quick BROCCOLI AND RICOTTA OMELET

Your omelet will be a glowing success if the filling is hot before you place it in the eggs. Also, make two omelets to better control the texture of the eggs.

2 cups tiny broccoli florets

½ cup part-skim ricotta cheese

1 tablespoon minced fresh basil, or ½ teaspoon dried

2 tablespoons grated Parmesan cheese

Salt

Freshly ground pepper

Butter for greasing

4 eggs, well beaten

Serves 2

1 In a medium-size saucepan, steam the broccoli in a vegetable steamer or with just a little bit of water until it is tender yet still bright green, about 5 minutes. Taste to see if it is cooked properly. If it is too crunchy, cook a few minutes more. Drain thoroughly and return to the pot.

2 In a small bowl, combine the ricotta, basil, Parmesan cheese, and salt and pepper to taste. Gently stir into the broccoli. Cover the pot and keep warm over low heat.

3 Lightly coat an omelet pan with some butter and heat the pan over medium-high heat. Pour in half the eggs and stir with a fork until curds begin to form. Shake the pan a little to distribute the liquid. When the omelet begins to set but is still slightly wet, spoon on half the hot broccoli mixture. Immediately fold over the omelet and serve. Repeat with the remaining eggs and filling.

Quick ZUCCHINI, CHEDDAR, AND SALSA OMELET

Here's a tasty omelet
that can be easily put together at a moment's
notice. Cooked rice is a suitable side dish.

2 teaspoons olive oil

2 cups thinly sliced
zucchini (from 2 small
zucchini, quartered
lengthwise and thinly
sliced)

½ teaspoon dried oregano

¼ cup mild or medium
salsa (homemade or store-
bought)

Freshly ground black
pepper

Butter for greasing

4 eggs, well beaten

1 cup (3 ounces) grated
Cheddar cheese

Serves 2

1 Heat the oil in a small skillet over medium heat. Add the zucchini and oregano and sauté until almost tender, about 5 minutes. Stir in the salsa and black pepper and cook until the zucchini is tender, not crunchy or mushy. The mixture should not be watery at this point. If there is any liquid, raise the heat and boil to evaporate. Keep the zucchini hot on low heat while you make the omelet.

2 Lightly grease an omelet pan with some butter and heat the pan over medium-high heat. When it is hot, pour in half the beaten eggs. Stir the eggs with a fork just until curds begin to form. Tip the pan slightly to cause the liquid eggs to run to the sides. Cook until set but slightly wet, about 1 minute total.

3 Place half the cheese on one side of the omelet. Spoon on half the zucchini mixture, then flip the omelet over to cover it. Slide the omelet onto a serving plate. Repeat to make another omelet.

Quick SZECHUAN CABBAGE AND MUSHROOMS IN CHILI SAUCE

When I want a low-fat dish with a lot of kick, I inevitably turn to spicy Chinese food. Serve this with rice (cook about 1 cup), which should be completely cooked and kept warm on the back burner when you begin stir-frying.

THE SAUCE

1½ teaspoons cornstarch

1 teaspoon water

1 tablespoon chili paste with garlic

3 tablespoons tamari soy sauce

¼ cup Chinese rice wine or dry sherry

1 teaspoon sugar

....

2-pound head napa (Chinese) cabbage

2 tablespoons vegetable or peanut oil

4 cups (about 12 ounces) sliced mushrooms

2 scallions, very thinly sliced

Serves 3

1 Stir the cornstarch and water together in a small bowl. Stir in all the remaining sauce ingredients and set aside.

2 Chop the root end off the cabbage and discard. Wash the leaves thoroughly. Chop the cabbage into 1½-inch pieces. It should yield 8 to 10 cups.

3 Heat the oil over medium-high heat in a wok or large skillet until hot but not smoking. Add the mushrooms and stir-fry until brown and juicy, about 5 minutes. Raise the heat to high. Add the cabbage and stir-fry, using 2 spoons or spatulas to toss it, for about 3 minutes, just until it wilts.

4 Stir the sauce once more. Pour onto the vegetables. Sprinkle on the scallions. Toss a few seconds, or until the sauce thickens. Serve on rice.

STUFFED ZUCCHINI WITH CHUNKY TOMATO SAUCE

*S*tuffed vegetables make
*a very attractive and satisfying main course.
Serve these stuffed zucchini with buttered egg
noodles for a good match.*

4 medium zucchini

1 tablespoon unsalted butter, cut into bits

Salt

Freshly ground pepper

2 tablespoons olive oil

2 garlic cloves, minced

1 medium onion, finely chopped

1 egg, beaten

½ cup diced roasted red peppers (from a 7-ounce jar)

¼ cup minced fresh parsley

1 cup bread crumbs

1 cup grated Swiss or Cheddar cheese

1 tablespoon minced fresh basil, or ½ teaspoon dried

½ teaspoon dried oregano

THE SAUCE

1 tablespoon olive oil

1 medium onion, finely diced

2 cups canned plum tomatoes, finely chopped,

1 Cut the ends off the zucchini. Halve lengthwise, then with a teaspoon carefully scoop out their centers, leaving a ¼-inch-thick wall. Finely chop the centers and set aside. Place the zucchini boats in a large skillet (you will have to do this in batches) with ½ inch of water. Cover the pan and bring it to a boil. Cook about 5 minutes, or until the zucchini are tender but not at all mushy. Place them on a cotton kitchen towel to drain.

2 Lightly oil a baking dish large enough to hold the zucchini. Place them in the dish, cavity side up, then sprinkle the butter bits in the shells. Season with salt and pepper to taste.

3 Drain the water and wipe the skillet dry. Pour in the oil and heat over medium heat. Add the garlic and onion and sauté until the onion is tender, about 10 minutes. Add the chopped zucchini and sauté about 10 minutes more, or until the zucchini is just tender. Scrape into a large bowl.

4 Mix in the egg, roasted peppers, parsley, bread crumbs, cheese, basil, oregano, and salt and pepper to taste. Stuff the zucchini boats with the mixture, carefully pressing it down to make it compact.

with their juice

Salt

Freshly ground pepper

Serves 4

5 Preheat the oven to 375 degrees.

6 Bake the zucchini, uncovered, for 30 minutes, or until golden brown and sizzling.

7 Meanwhile, make the sauce. Heat the olive oil in a medium-size skillet. Add the onion and sauté until tender, about 10 minutes. Stir in the tomatoes along with salt and pepper to taste. Cook, stirring occasionally, until the sauce begins to thicken, about 10 minutes. Put a few spoonfuls of sauce in the center of each serving plate and spread it out. Place the stuffed zucchini on the sauce.

∾ Note: May be prepared through step 4 up to 24 hours in advance and refrigerated. Bring to room temperature before baking.

SPICED CAULIFLOWER WITH FRAGRANT RICE PILAF

Here are two Indian
dishes that complement each other with a
mélange of spicy, tangy, hot, and sweet flavors.
A few spoonfuls of plain yogurt on the side add
a soothing touch and a delightful contrast.

THE PILAF

1 tablespoon vegetable oil

1 onion, diced

1 cup basmati or converted rice

2 cloves

1 cinnamon stick

1 bay leaf

¼ teaspoon ground cardamom

¼ cup sliced almonds

⅓ cup raisins

½ teaspoon salt

2 cups water

THE CAULIFLOWER

2 tablespoons vegetable oil

1 large onion, diced

2 garlic cloves, minced

½ teaspoon minced fresh ginger

1 teaspoon ground coriander seed

1 teaspoon turmeric

½ teaspoon ground cumin

1 In a medium-size saucepan, heat the oil over medium heat. Add the onion and sauté for 5 minutes. Stir in all the remaining pilaf ingredients except the water and cook 2 minutes more, stirring often.

2 Pour in the water, cover the pot, then bring to a boil. Lower the heat to a simmer and cook over low heat until all the water is absorbed, about 20 minutes.

3 Meanwhile, make the cauliflower. Heat the oil in a large skillet over medium heat. Add the onion, garlic, and ginger and sauté for 5 minutes, tossing often. Stir in all of the spices and cook for 2 minutes, again stirring often.

4 Add the tomatoes; cook 2 minutes. Thoroughly mix in the cauliflower and salt and cover the pan. Cook, stirring occasionally, until the cauliflower is tender, about 7 minutes. Remove the cover. (If the sauce is watery, cook at high heat for a few seconds until it thickens.) Stir in the peas and cilantro and cook 1 minute more.

5 Return to the rice pilaf. When all the water is absorbed and the rice is tender, remove the cinnamon stick and bay leaf, then fluff the rice with a fork. Let sit, covered, for 2 minutes before serving. Serve the rice alongside the cauliflower.

¼ teaspoon ground
cardamom

⅛ teaspoon cayenne, or
more to taste

1½ cups finely chopped
canned tomatoes, with
their juice

1 medium cauliflower, cut
into small florets (about
6 cups)

¼ teaspoon salt

1 cup frozen peas, thawed

1 tablespoon minced
cilantro or fresh parsley

Serves 4

PIZZAS, CALZONES, FOCACCE, AND BOBOLI

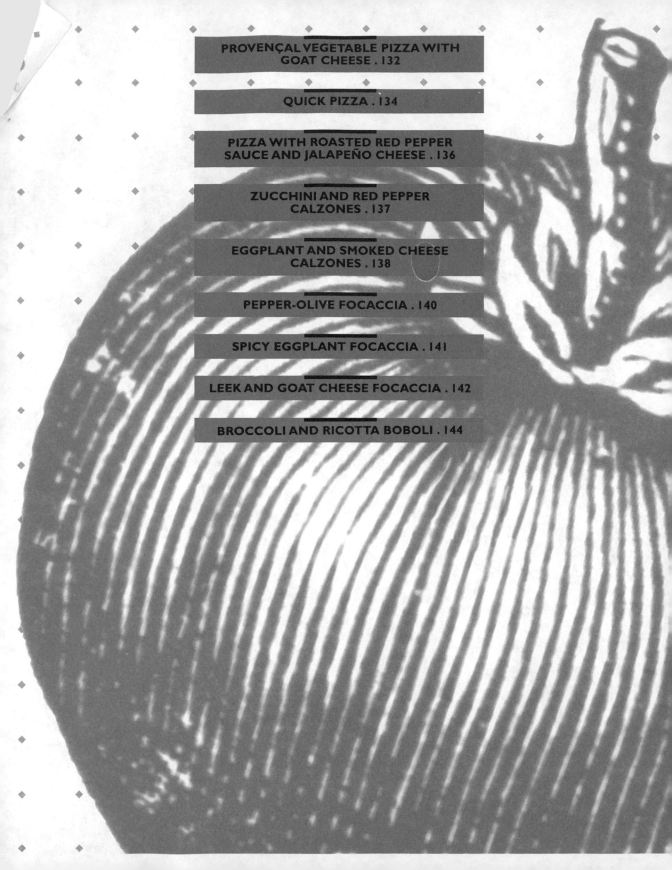

To my mind, pizza and its relatives are superlative foods. With a crisp, well-made crust as a base, they become ideal vehicles for combining your favorite cheeses, vegetables, and herbs.

A calzone is actually a pizza folded over to make a turnover. These self-contained stuffed pouches can be made any size, so if you want party food that's easy to eat, you can make them smaller than my recipes suggest.

Focaccia (pronounced fo-KAH-cha) is another cousin to pizza. Its thicker, often herb-laced crust can be lightly dressed with just a sprinkling of Parmesan cheese and served as one would serve bread, or it can be covered with a more substantial topping and made into a meal, as I have done here. I have gotten great results using frozen bread dough as a quick and easy base for focaccia. Seek out a good-quality dough, additive-free and containing just flour, water, yeast, and salt.

To incorporate herbs and oil in a thawed dough, make sure your dough is at room temperature, then knead in the added ingredients as best you can. Let the dough rest 10 minutes or so, then knead again until evenly blended.

If you want to make your focaccia dough from scratch, follow the recipe for pizza dough (page 132), using 1 tablespoon oil in the dough; omit incorporating more oil in the dough if the recipe calls for it.

PROVENÇAL VEGETABLE PIZZA WITH GOAT CHEESE

This is a fabulous pizza—both to look at and to savor. First, a layer of cheese is sprinkled on the dough, then a very garlicky tomato-zucchini mixture, and finally spoonfuls of creamy goat cheese. It's easy to make, and becomes even easier if the zucchini mixture is made early in the day.

THE DOUGH

1 cup warm water

2 teaspoons active dry yeast

½ teaspoon sugar

2 tablespoons olive oil

2½ cups unbleached flour

1 teaspoon salt

....

Oil for greasing bowl and pizza pans

THE TOPPING

2 tablespoons olive oil

6 garlic cloves, minced

¼ teaspoon crushed red pepper flakes

6 cups thinly sliced zucchini (from 3 medium zucchini, quartered lengthwise and thinly sliced)

1 teaspoon dried oregano

2 tablespoons shredded fresh basil, or 1 teaspoon dried

1 To make the dough, combine the water, yeast, and sugar in a small bowl and stir to mix. Let sit 10 minutes. Stir in the olive oil.

2 Combine the flour and salt in a large bowl. Pour in the yeast mixture and stir until a ball of dough is formed. Turn onto a floured surface and knead until smooth, about 5 minutes.

3 Very lightly oil a large glass or ceramic bowl. Place the ball of dough in it, rotating the dough so the entire ball is oiled. Cover the bowl with plastic wrap and put in a warm place until the dough rises to double its size, 1 to 1½ hours. (Sometimes I heat my oven for a minute—just until it is warm, not hot—then turn it off and place the bowl in the oven.)

4 Meanwhile, make the topping. Heat the olive oil in a large skillet over medium-high heat. Add the garlic and red pepper flakes and sauté for 2 minutes. Stir in the zucchini, oregano, dried basil (if using fresh basil, see step 9), thyme, salt, and ground pepper. Sauté until the zucchini is tender but not mushy, about 10 minutes.

¼ teaspoon dried thyme

Salt

Generous seasoning of freshly ground pepper

½ cup canned crushed tomatoes

10 oil-cured olives, pitted and quartered (see note, page 25)

....

3 cups (9 ounces) grated part-skim mozzarella cheese

6 ounces goat cheese

Serves 4 to 6 (1 17 × 11-inch pizza or 2 9-inch pizzas)

5 Mix in the crushed tomatoes and olives and cook 2 minutes more. Remove from the heat and let cool. (The vegetable mixture can be made and kept refrigerated for up to 24 hours in advance. Bring to room temperature before assembling the pizza.)

6 Preheat the oven to 450 degrees. Lightly oil a 17 × 11-inch baking sheet or 2 9-inch pizza pans.

7 When the dough has doubled its size, punch it down to its original size and remove all the air bubbles. (If you are not ready to cook the pizza, chill the dough.) Roll the dough to fit the pans or baking sheet, stretching the edges as necessary once in the pan.

8 Sprinkle on the mozzarella cheese. Spread the zucchini mixture evenly over the cheese.

9 Bake the pizza for 17 minutes, or until the crust is golden underneath. (Use a spatula to help you peek.) If you are using fresh basil, sprinkle it on the pizza now. Place small spoonfuls or chunks of goat cheese evenly over the pizza and bake 2 additional minutes. Slide the pizza onto a large cutting board and cut it into squares. Serve immediately.

QUICK PIZZA

Quick

This alternative to a yeast pizza dough is delicious. A delicate, crisp crust is created with baking powder as the leavener, making it ultraquick to prepare and lending itself to a variety of imaginative toppings. Below are some of my favorite choices. Feel free to improvise.

Oil for greasing pan

THE DOUGH

2 cups unbleached flour

½ cup whole wheat flour

1½ teaspoons baking powder

½ teaspoon salt

4 tablespoons unsalted butter, chilled and cut into pieces

1 cup low-fat milk

TOPPING SUGGESTIONS

Sliced tomatoes, grated Muenster and mozzarella cheeses (or crumbled Gorgonzola), topped with dried basil and oregano

Grated mozzarella cheese and strips of roasted red peppers, then gobs of goat cheese and shredded fresh basil once removed from the oven

Grated fontina cheese, then diced tomatoes, minced garlic, and cooked broccoli bits, with little spoonfuls of ricotta cheese all over the top, finally sprinkled with dried basil

1 Preheat the oven to 450 degrees. Lightly oil 2 17-inch-long baking sheets.

2 Place the two flours, baking powder, and salt in the container of a food processor and pulse until mixed. Drop in the butter pieces and pulse until large crumbs form. With the motor running, pour in the milk and process just until a clump of dough forms. (Alternatively, combine the dry ingredients in a large bowl. Add the butter pieces and rub into the flour with your fingertips until coarse crumbs form. Pour in the milk and stir just until combined.)

3 Scrape the dough onto a lightly floured surface. Gather it into 4 balls. Roll out each ball with a lightly floured rolling pin into an 8-inch circle. Place two circles on each prepared baking sheet.

4 Top with the toppings of your choice and bake 12 to 15 minutes, or until golden on top and bottom. Peek underneath the crust to make sure it is golden brown.

Grated Jarlsberg cheese, sautéed mushrooms, and minced garlic sprinkled all over

Grated Muenster cheese topped with sliced cherry tomatoes and little spoonfuls of pesto

Tomato sauce, chopped cilantro, spoonfuls of goat cheese, then grated Parmesan cheese sprinkled all over

Serves 4 (4 8-inch pizzas)

PIZZA WITH ROASTED RED PEPPER SAUCE AND JALAPEÑO CHEESE

No tomatoes on this pizza—the incomparable flavors of roasted red peppers and basil make up the delectable sauce, and the jalapeños give the pizza some kick without being overbearing.

Pizza dough (page 132)

....

1 7-ounce jar roasted red peppers, thoroughly drained and patted dry

2 garlic cloves, minced

2 tablespoons olive oil

½ teaspoon dried basil

Dash of cayenne

....

1½ cups (4½ ounces) grated Monterey Jack cheese with jalapeño peppers

1½ cups (4½ ounces) grated part-skim mozzarella cheese

Serves 4 (1 17 × 11-inch pizza or 2 9-inch pizzas)

1 While the pizza dough rises, make the sauce. Combine the roasted peppers, garlic, olive oil, basil, and cayenne in a blender or food processor and purée. Scrape it into a bowl.

2 Preheat the oven to 450 degrees. Lightly oil a baking sheet or pizza pans and proceed to line them as in step 7, page 133.

3 Spread the red pepper sauce on the dough. Sprinkle the two cheeses evenly over the dough. Bake 15 minutes, or until the crust is golden underneath.

ZUCCHINI AND RED PEPPER CALZONES

Crunchy pine nuts enhance this aromatic filling, adding both texture and flavor. Remember these calzones for a special luncheon; they'll be a big hit.

THE FILLING

1 tablespoon olive oil

4 garlic cloves, minced

2 medium zucchini, quartered lengthwise and thinly sliced (4 cups sliced)

1 red bell pepper, diced

1½ tablespoons pine nuts

½ cup tomato sauce (homemade or store-bought)

Freshly ground black pepper to taste

....

Pizza dough (page 132), or 1 pound frozen bread dough, thawed

½ pound thinly sliced or 2½ cups grated Muenster cheese

1 egg, beaten with 1 teaspoon water (egg wash)

Serves 4 to 6 (6 7 inch calzones)

1 Heat the oil in a large skillet over medium-high heat. Add the garlic and cook 1 minute. Stir in the zucchini, red pepper, and pine nuts. Sauté until the vegetables are tender yet still slightly crisp, about 7 minutes. Stir in the tomato sauce, season with the black pepper, then cook 1 minute more. Remove from the heat and let cool completely. The filling can be made up to 24 hours in advance and chilled. Bring to room temperature before using.

2 If you are making the dough from scratch, prepare the pizza dough as directed. After it has risen, punch it down and knead it a few times. If you are using purchased bread dough, go to the next step.

3 Preheat the oven to 375 degrees.

4 Continue with steps 5, 6, and 7 on pages 138 and 139 (Eggplant and Smoked Cheese Calzones).

EGGPLANT AND SMOKED CHEESE CALZONES

These folded pizzas are not difficult to make and are especially easy if you make the filling early in the day. If you are in a hurry, you can use a 1-pound package of store-bought frozen pizza or bread dough, thaw it, and proceed with step 5.

THE FILLING

1 tablespoon olive oil

1 medium onion, finely diced

2 garlic cloves, minced

1 16-ounce can tomatoes, finely chopped and drained, or 2 medium tomatoes, cored, seeded, and finely chopped

1 medium (1 pound) eggplant, peeled and finely diced

1 green pepper, cored and finely diced

½ teaspoon dried oregano

½ teaspoon salt

½ teaspoon sugar

Generous seasoning of freshly ground pepper

1 teaspoon balsamic or red wine vinegar

....

Pizza dough (page 132), or 1 pound frozen bread dough, thawed

2½ cups (about 8 ounces) grated smoked Gouda or

1 Heat the oil in a large skillet over medium heat. Add the onion and garlic and sauté, tossing often, until the onion is very tender, about 10 minutes.

2 Stir in all the remaining filling ingredients. Cover the pan and cook for 15 minutes, or until the eggplant is very tender. Stir occasionally. Remove the cover and cook away any juices that may have accumulated. Remove from the heat and let cool. The filling may be prepared and chilled up to 24 hours in advance. Bring to room temperature before using.

3 If making the dough from scratch, prepare the pizza dough as directed. After it has risen, punch it down and knead it a few times.

4 Preheat the oven to 375 degrees.

5 Divide the dough into 6 pieces, then roll each piece into a ball. With a rolling pin, flatten one ball into a 6- or 7-inch circle. Place a small cup of water beside you, dip your finger into the water, and moisten the outer edges of the circle. Place a sixth of the eggplant filling on half of the circle, then top with a sixth of the grated cheese. Fold the dough over the filling to make a turnover or half-moon shape. Pinch and roll the edges closed.

smoked mozzarella cheese

1 egg, beaten with
1 teaspoon water (egg
wash)

*Serves 4 to 6 (6 7-inch
calzones)*

6 With a pastry brush, lightly brush the top of the calzone with some of the beaten egg wash. Place on an oiled baking sheet, then make 5 more calzones. (You will probably need two baking sheets. In this case, bake on two oven racks, then switch halfway through cooking.)

7 Bake 25 minutes, or until golden brown. Let sit at least 20 minutes before serving. They should be served warm, not piping hot.

Note: Leftover calzones can be refrigerated and reheated a few days later; they'll still be great.

Quick PEPPER-OLIVE FOCACCIA

Rosemary-flecked dough makes a savory bed for a Mediterranean-style mélange of peppers and olives. This focaccia is my favorite.

1 tablespoon olive oil

4 garlic cloves, minced

1 large red bell pepper, thinly sliced into strips

1 large green bell pepper, thinly sliced into strips

8 oil-cured or 6 kalamata olives, pitted and sliced (see note, page 25)

....

1 pound frozen bread dough, thawed and at room temperature

½ teaspoon dried rosemary, crumbled

Generous seasoning of freshly ground pepper

2 tablespoons olive oil

½ cup plus 2 tablespoons grated Parmesan cheese

Serves 4

1 Heat the oil in a large skillet over medium heat. Add the garlic and cook 1 minute. Do not let it brown. Mix in the peppers and cook, stirring often, until very tender, about 10 minutes. Remove from the heat and stir in the olives. Let cool.

2 Place the thawed dough in a large bowl. Sprinkle on the rosemary, pepper, and 1 tablespoon of the olive oil; knead these into the dough until incorporated.

3 Preheat the oven to 400 degrees.

4 Roll and stretch the dough into a 9 × 12-inch rectangle, then place on a baking sheet. Spread the remaining tablespoon of olive oil all over the surface of the dough. Sprinkle on ½ cup of the cheese, then pat it down with your hand to help it adhere.

5 Place in the oven and bake until the cheese is a rich golden brown, about 12 minutes. Remove from the oven and spread the peppers all over the focaccia. Sprinkle on the remaining 2 tablespoons of cheese. Bake 7 more minutes. Cut into 4 squares and serve.

Quick SPICY EGGPLANT FOCACCIA

he crust in this focaccia develops a nutty flavor by having part of the Parmesan cheese kneaded into the dough before baking. For best flavor, serve this one warm rather than hot.

2 tablespoons olive oil

4 garlic cloves, minced

½ teaspoon crushed red pepper flakes

1 small (¾ pound) eggplant, peeled and cut into ½-inch dice

1 small green pepper, cut into ½-inch dice

1 cup tomato sauce, homemade or store-bought

½ teaspoon dried basil

2 teaspoons water

Salt

Freshly ground pepper

....

1 pound frozen bread dough, thawed and at room temperature

5 tablespoons grated Parmesan cheese

Flour for dusting

Serves 4

1 Heat the oil in a large skillet over medium heat. Add the garlic and red pepper flakes and cook for 1 minute, stirring constantly.

2 Stir in the eggplant, green pepper, tomato sauce, basil, water, and salt and pepper to taste. Cover the pan and cook, stirring occasionally, 15 to 20 minutes, or until the eggplant and pepper are tender and not at all crunchy. Because there isn't much liquid in this mixture, it will "steam" rather than simmer. Remove from the heat and let cool.

3 Preheat the oven to 400 degrees.

4 Place the thawed dough in a large bowl. Sprinkle on 2 tablespoons of the cheese and knead it into the dough. Roll the dough into a 9 × 12-inch rectangle, flouring the work surface as necessary. Place it on a baking sheet.

5 Bake the dough 10 minutes. Remove from the oven, then spread the eggplant mixture all over the dough. Sprinkle the remaining 3 tablespoons of Parmesan cheese on top of the eggplant.

6 Bake 10 more minutes, or until the dough is golden brown. Place the focaccia on a cutting board and cut into squares. Let cool about 15 minutes, serving it warm, not hot.

Quick LEEK AND GOAT CHEESE FOCACCIA

Madeleine Kamman, on her first-rate cooking show **Madeleine Cooks,** once used a combination of leeks, walnuts, and goat cheese on a pizza and thus inspired me to try it here. It is a fabulous medley of flavors, making a memorable focaccia. Don't hesitate to pack it for a picnic; it is delicious at room temperature.

2 medium-large leeks

2 teaspoons plus 1 tablespoon olive oil

¼ cup heavy cream

Salt

Freshly ground pepper

1 pound frozen bread dough, thawed and at room temperature

½ teaspoon dried thyme

Flour for dusting

2 tablespoons finely chopped walnuts

4 ounces garlic and herb or plain goat cheese, cut into small pieces

Serves 4

1 To clean the leeks, make a vertical slit in each along its length through to the back. Rinse under cold running water, flipping through the leaves with your fingers to rid them of all sand and dirt. Thinly slice the leeks, using as much green as possible, but avoiding the extra-thick outer leaves.

2 Heat the 2 teaspoons of olive oil in a medium-size skillet over medium heat. Add the leeks and sauté until tender, about 10 minutes. Add the cream and salt and pepper to taste and cook 2 minutes more, or just until the cream thickens.

3 Preheat the oven to 400 degrees.

4 Place the thawed dough in a large bowl. Evenly sprinkle on the thyme, then the remaining tablespoon of olive oil. Knead until incorporated. You can let it rest after a few minutes of kneading and it will absorb some oil, then knead a bit more. Roll the dough into a 9 × 12-inch rectangle, flouring the work surface as necessary to prevent sticking. Place the dough on a baking sheet.

5 Bake the dough 10 minutes. Remove from the oven, then spread the leeks all over the dough to within ½ inch of the edges. Sprinkle on the walnuts. Bake 10 more minutes. Remove from the oven and drop on the pieces of goat cheese. Bake 3 additional minutes, or until golden. Let cool a few minutes before serving. Serve cut into squares.

Quick BROCCOLI AND RICOTTA BOBOLI

Purchasing a premade boboli (cheese crust) makes this a snap to prepare.

1 tablespoon olive oil

4 garlic cloves, minced

4 cups tiny broccoli florets (from 1 small bunch broccoli)

⅓ cup water

2 scallions, very thinly sliced

Salt

Generous seasoning of freshly ground pepper

1 cup part-skim ricotta cheese

2 tablespoons chopped fresh basil, or 1 teaspoon dried

1 large (1 pound) boboli

1 cup grated part-skim mozzarella cheese

Serves 4

1 Heat the oil in a large skillet over medium heat. Add the garlic and sauté 2 minutes. Stir in the broccoli and toss to coat with the garlic. Pour in the water and cover the pan. Steam the broccoli until tender, still bright green but not crunchy, about 7 minutes.

2 Remove the cover and stir in the scallions, salt, and pepper. Cook until all the liquid has evaporated, just a few more minutes. Set aside to cool.

3 Preheat the oven to 450 degrees.

4 Combine the ricotta and basil in a small bowl. Spread it on the boboli, then place the boboli on a baking sheet. Spoon the broccoli all over the top; cover with the mozzarella cheese.

5 Bake 10 to 12 minutes, or until the crust is golden and the cheese is sizzling. Cut into 8 wedges.

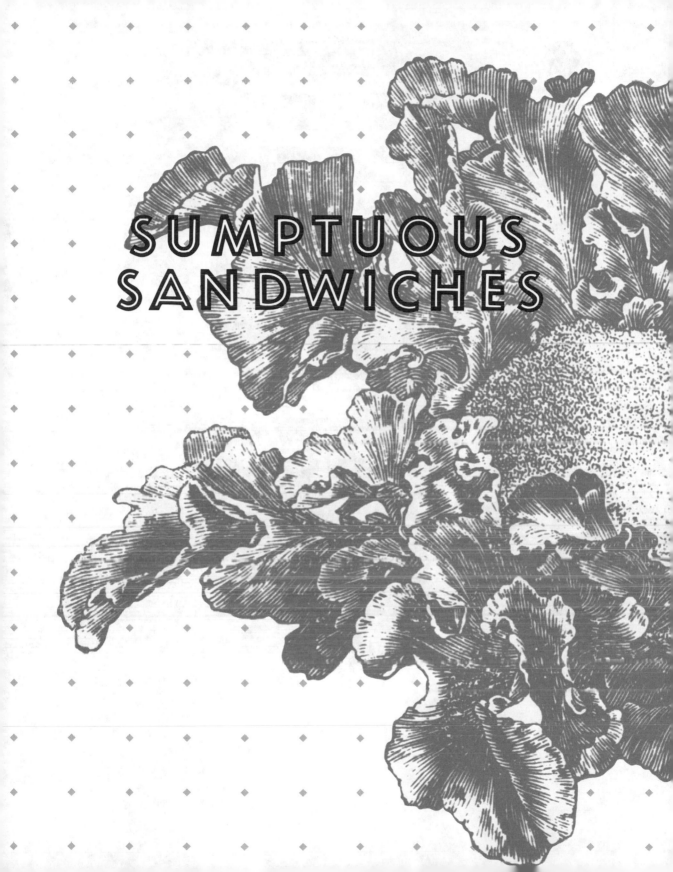

SUMPTUOUS SANDWICHES

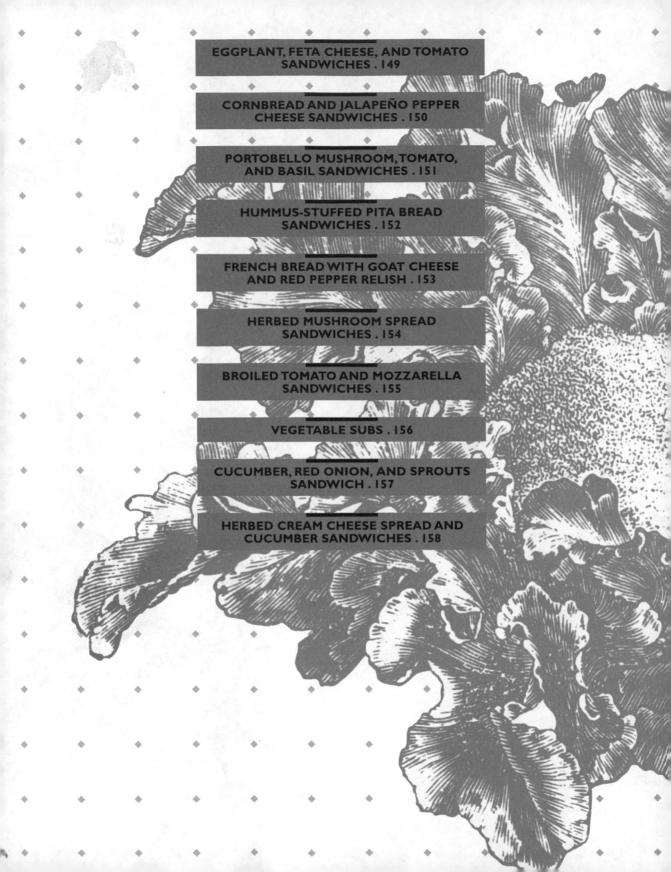

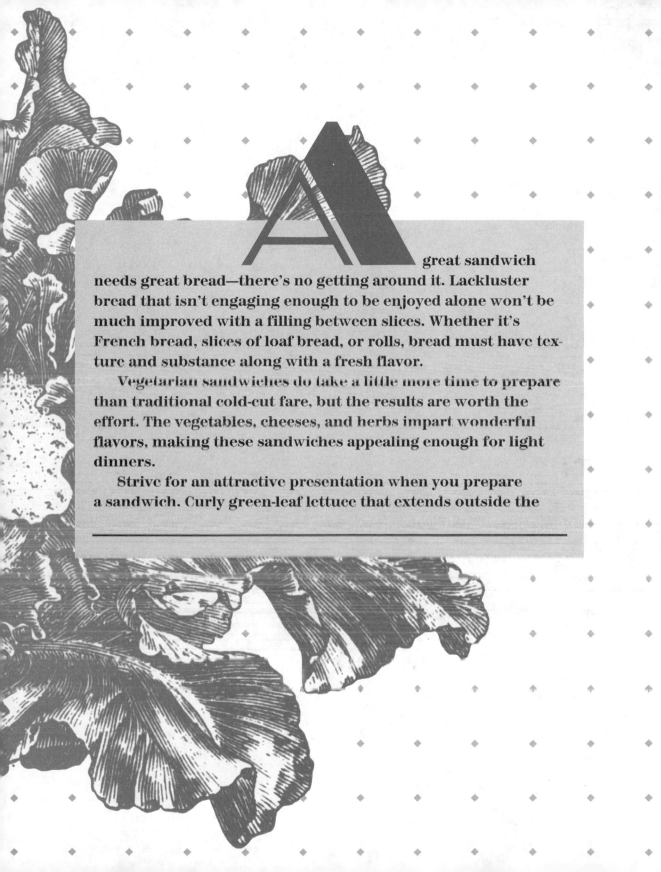

great sandwich needs great bread—there's no getting around it. Lackluster bread that isn't engaging enough to be enjoyed alone won't be much improved with a filling between slices. Whether it's French bread, slices of loaf bread, or rolls, bread must have texture and substance along with a fresh flavor.

Vegetarian sandwiches do take a little more time to prepare than traditional cold-cut fare, but the results are worth the effort. The vegetables, cheeses, and herbs impart wonderful flavors, making these sandwiches appealing enough for light dinners.

Strive for an attractive presentation when you prepare a sandwich. Curly green-leaf lettuce that extends outside the

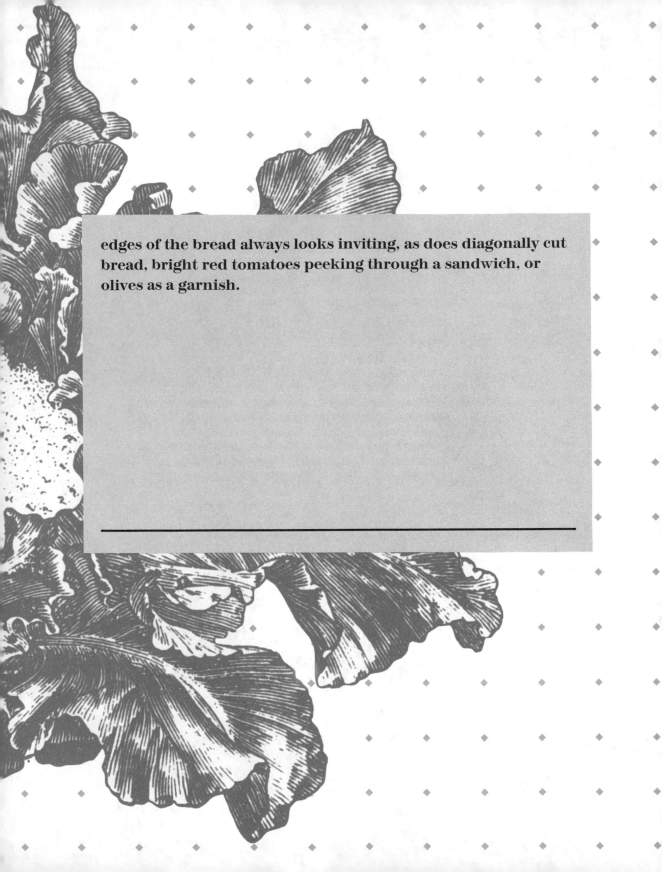

edges of the bread always looks inviting, as does diagonally cut bread, bright red tomatoes peeking through a sandwich, or olives as a garnish.

EGGPLANT, FETA CHEESE, AND TOMATO SANDWICHES

Layered with
fresh basil, this sandwich's outstanding flavor
will please you for days.

¼ cup bread crumbs
(approximately)

1 medium (1 pound)
eggplant, skin left on and
cut into ¼-inch slices

7 tablespoons olive oil

1 loaf French bread or
crusty peasant bread

Freshly ground pepper

4 ounces feta cheese, thinly
sliced

2 medium tomatoes, thinly
sliced

16 fresh basil leaves

Serves 4

1 Preheat the broiler. Place the bread crumbs on a small plate. Brush both sides of each eggplant slice with oil, using 3 tablespoons in all. Press both sides of the eggplant into the bread crumbs, then place on a baking sheet. Broil until golden brown, turn, and brown the other side. Set the eggplant aside to cool.

2 Cut the bread in half horizontally so the crust makes up the top and bottom of each sandwich. Cut the loaf into 4 portions.

3 To assemble each sandwich, drizzle 1 tablespoon of the olive oil on the inside of the bread, then season generously with pepper. Place a quarter of the feta cheese slices on the bread, top with a quarter of the tomato slices, tear up 4 basil leaves into small pieces and sprinkle them on the tomato, then place a few eggplant slices on top. Cover with the top of the bread and slice the sandwich in half.

CORNBREAD AND JALAPEÑO PEPPER CHEESE SANDWICHES

Here is a simple idea for a sandwich that works well because the foods it combines—cornbread and jalapeño pepper cheese—are perfectly compatible. Make the cornbread the night before or early in the morning so it has ample time to cool. The sandwiches can be served alone or accompanied by some marinated vegetables or lightly tossed greens.

THE CORNBREAD

Butter for greasing

¾ cup unbleached white flour

¼ cup whole wheat flour

1 cup cornmeal

1 tablespoon baking powder

½ teaspoon salt

¼ cup sugar

1 egg, beaten

1¼ cups low-fat milk

3 tablespoons butter, melted and cooled

....

8 ounces (brick) Monterey Jack cheese with jalapeño peppers, thinly sliced (about 32 slices)

Serves 6 to 8

1 Preheat the oven to 400 degrees (375 degrees if your baking dish is glass). Butter a 12 × 7 × 2-inch baking pan or dish (see note) and set aside.

2 In a large bowl, combine the two flours, cornmeal, baking powder, salt, and sugar.

3 Thoroughly combine the egg, milk, and melted butter in another bowl. Pour this mixture into the dry ingredients and stir just until blended. Do not overbeat. Scrape into the prepared pan and bake 20 to 25 minutes, or until golden on top. Cool completely on a wire rack.

4 Cut the cornbread into 16 pieces about 2 × 3 inches. Cut each piece in half horizontally, then place a few thin slices of cheese on each bottom half. Cover with the top slice of bread to make small sandwiches.

Note: This makes a low cornbread, suitable for sandwiches. If you want to make it to serve plain rather than in sandwiches, use an 8 × 8-inch pan and cook 25 minutes.

PORTOBELLO MUSHROOM, TOMATO, AND BASIL SANDWICHES

*Y*ou can grill these giant
Portobello mushrooms instead of sautéing
them by removing the stems and brushing both
sides with olive oil. Grill them about 3 minutes
on each side. Whether you sauté or grill
them, you'll have a knockout of a sandwich.

4 tablespoons olive oil

8 ounces Portobello
mushrooms, sliced ½-inch
thick

2 teaspoons balsamic
vinegar

1 small garlic clove,
pressed or minced

3 7-inch pieces narrow
French bread, each sliced
horizontally

6 tomato slices, each cut in
half

9 basil leaves

Salt

Freshly ground pepper

Serves 3

1 Heat 1 tablespoon of the olive oil in a large
skillet over medium heat. Add the mushrooms
and sauté until brown and juicy, about 10 minutes.

2 Meanwhile, in a small dish combine the
remaining 3 tablespoons oil with the vinegar and
garlic and stir to blend.

3 If the French bread isn't absolutely fresh and
crisp, heat it in the oven a few minutes, until just
hot.

4 To assemble the sandwiches, spread ⅙ of the oil
and vinegar mixture on each half of French bread.
On each bottom half of the bread, layer ⅓ of the
mushrooms, tomato slices, and basil leaves.
Season with salt and pepper and top with the
remaining bread. Slice the sandwiches in half and
serve immediately.

HUMMUS-STUFFED PITA BREAD SANDWICHES

This sandwich has become almost standard fare on menus in vegetarian restaurants, and because it is so good when well made, I decided to include it here. When hummus is used as a spread, it should be thicker than the traditional dip consistency, so be cautious when adding the water to avoid making it too thin. Conversely, if you want to turn the leftover hummus spread into a dip, thin it with a little water.

1 cup cooked chickpeas (either home-cooked or rinsed canned chickpeas)

½ cup tahini

1 large garlic clove, minced

Juice of 1 lemon (3 to 4 tablespoons)

¼ teaspoon salt

¼ to ⅓ cup cold water

....

4 6-inch pita breads (see note)

Thinly sliced cucumber

Thinly sliced red onion

Thinly sliced tomato (optional)

Alfalfa sprouts or leaf lettuce

Serves 4

1 To make the hummus, combine the chickpeas, tahini, garlic, lemon juice, and salt in a food processor. Process until smooth. Slowly pour in ¼ cup water and process again. Check the consistency; it should be spreadable, not runny. Add more water if it is too thick. Scrape into a bowl.

2 Cut the pita breads in half to make two pockets. Heat in a toaster or oven just to soften. Let cool slightly.

3 Spread hummus in each pocket. Fill with some cucumber slices, red onion, tomato, and sprouts.

Note: This sandwich is also delicious on sliced whole grain bread.

FRENCH BREAD WITH GOAT CHEESE AND RED PEPPER RELISH

This winning combination can be turned into hors d'oeuvres by slicing the French bread into thin rounds and making a small version of this open-face sandwich.

1 tablespoon olive oil

2 medium onions, finely diced

2 red bell peppers, finely diced

1 teaspoon sugar

2 teaspoons balsamic or red wine vinegar

Salt

Generous seasoning of freshly ground pepper

½ to 1 teaspoon capers

....

1 loaf French bread

4 ounces goat cheese

Serves 4

1 To make the pepper relish, heat the oil in a large skillet over medium-high heat. Add the onions and sauté until tender and beginning to brown, about 10 minutes.

2 Stir in the peppers and cook 10 more minutes, stirring often. Mix in the sugar, vinegar, salt, and pepper. Reduce the heat to medium, cover the pan, and cook until the mixture is very soft and the juices are somewhat caramelized, not watery, about 20 more minutes. Stir occasionally.

3 Scrape the mixture into a bowl, then stir in the capers. Let cool completely; chill until ready to use. Bring the relish back to room temperature before serving.

4 Slice the French bread horizontally and cut into 3- to 4-inch lengths. Heat in a 400-degree oven until slightly crisp (not hard).

5 Spread some goat cheese on each piece, then top with a spoonful of the pepper relish.

HERBED MUSHROOM SPREAD SANDWICHES

*S*ucculent mushrooms
laced with herbs make a sumptuous base for
sandwiches. I especially like this spread on toast
made from a good-quality Vienna or Italian
bread.

2 teaspoons olive oil

12 ounces mushrooms, finely chopped (about 4 cups)

1 teaspoon tamari soy sauce

¼ teaspoon dried thyme

¼ teaspoon dried oregano

¼ teaspoon dried dill

Freshly ground pepper to taste

1 tablespoon mayonnaise, plus extra for spreading

1½ tablespoons very thinly sliced celery

6 slices bread (preferably Vienna or Italian)

3 pieces green leaf lettuce

Serves 3

1 Heat the oil in a large skillet over medium-high heat. Add the mushrooms and sauté them, tossing often, until their juices have been released and then evaporate, about 10 minutes.

2 Stir in the tamari, herbs, and pepper to taste and cook until the mushrooms begin to stick to the pan, about 2 minutes more. Scrape the mixture into a bowl and cool to room temperature. Stir in the tablespoon of mayonnaise and the celery and chill until ready to serve.

3 Lightly toast the bread. Spread each piece with a very thin layer of mayonnaise. Divide the mushrooms and spread on 3 of the bread slices. Top with the lettuce and remaining bread. Slice the sandwiches in half diagonally and serve.

BROILED TOMATO AND MOZZARELLA SANDWICHES

Quick

These open-face sand-wiches capture the fresh taste of the tomatoes and herbs with sweet mozzarella cheese as the perfect backdrop. Be certain to serve them right from the oven so the cheese stays soft.

French bread sliced horizontally, or slices of firm bread such as sourdough

Olive oil

Very thinly sliced part-skim mozzarella cheese

Thin tomato slices

Dried basil

Dried oregano

Freshly ground pepper

Grated Parmesan cheese

1 Preheat the broiler. Lightly toast whichever bread you choose, then brush the top of each piece with a little olive oil. Place the bread on a baking sheet.

2 Place a few slices of mozzarella cheese on the bread (you don't need much). Top with the tomato slices. Generously sprinkle basil, oregano, and pepper on the tomato. Sprinkle Parmesan cheese all over the tomato. Broil the sandwiches until the mozzarella is melted and bubbly and the Parmesan cheese has turned golden brown. Serve immediately.

Quick VEGETABLE SUBS

These submarine (hero) sandwiches are a staple in my family. We rely on them for lunch more than any other sandwich because they are so easy and so satisfying. The added bonus is that they are equally popular with any meat lover who joins us for lunch.

Submarine, grinder, or hero rolls

Vinaigrette salad dressing

Mayonnaise

Freshly ground black pepper

Thinly sliced Muenster, Swiss, or provolone cheese

Thinly sliced tomato

Thinly sliced red onion

Thinly sliced green or red bell pepper strips

Romaine or leaf lettuce

Optional additions: sliced black olives, sliced pickles, sliced pickled peppers

1 Slice the rolls almost all the way through. Heat them briefly in a 350-degree oven if they are not perfectly fresh.

2 Open the rolls and spread a very thin coating of vinaigrette on each half, then top with a thin layer of mayonnaise and some black pepper. Layer all the remaining ingredients on the rolls, being careful not to overstuff them. Close the sandwiches and slice in half.

Quick CUCUMBER, RED ONION, AND SPROUTS SANDWICH

Here is another sandwich that I frequently serve my family. It is especially convenient because we always seem to have the ingredients on hand. This trio of vegetables works well together, and it is enhanced in a sandwich made with whole grain toast, although other breads such as crusty rolls work well, too. If you are not an onion lover, just omit it and you'll still have a delicious sandwich.

Sliced whole wheat or sourdough bread

Mayonnaise

Cucumber, peeled and cut into ⅓-inch slices

Freshly ground black pepper

Red onion, very thinly sliced

Alfalfa sprouts

Toast the bread. Spread with some mayonnaise. Layer on the cucumber, black pepper, onion, and sprouts. Top with slices of toast to make sandwiches. Slice in half diagonally and serve.

HERBED CREAM CHEESE SPREAD AND CUCUMBER SANDWICHES

Quick

*Y*ou can certainly exper-
iment with different combinations of herbs, but
my favorite mixture is the one below where
the flavors blend and none is too overpowering.

8 ounces Neufchâtel (light cream cheese), at room temperature

1½ tablespoons low-fat milk

2 scallions, very thinly sliced, or 3 tablespoons very finely chopped red onion

2 tablespoons minced fresh parsley

1 teaspoon minced fresh dill, or ¼ teaspoon dried

1 teaspoon minced fresh thyme, or ¼ teaspoon dried

1 teaspoon minced fresh basil, or ¼ teaspoon dried

Generous seasoning of freshly ground pepper

Dash of salt

8 slices whole grain bread

1 cucumber, peeled and cut into ¼-inch slices

Serves 4

1 In a large bowl, work the cream cheese and milk together with a fork until blended, then beat it until smooth. Stir in the scallions, herbs, pepper, and salt. Cover and chill at least 1 hour for the flavors to meld.

2 To make each sandwich, spread the mixture on both slices of bread and place the cucumber slices in between.

BREAKFAST AND BRUNCH

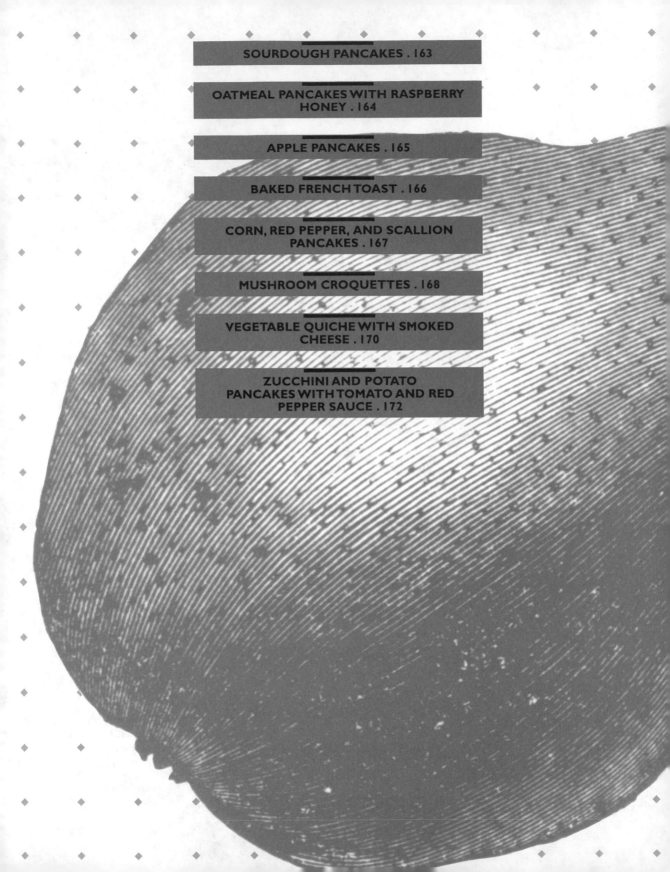

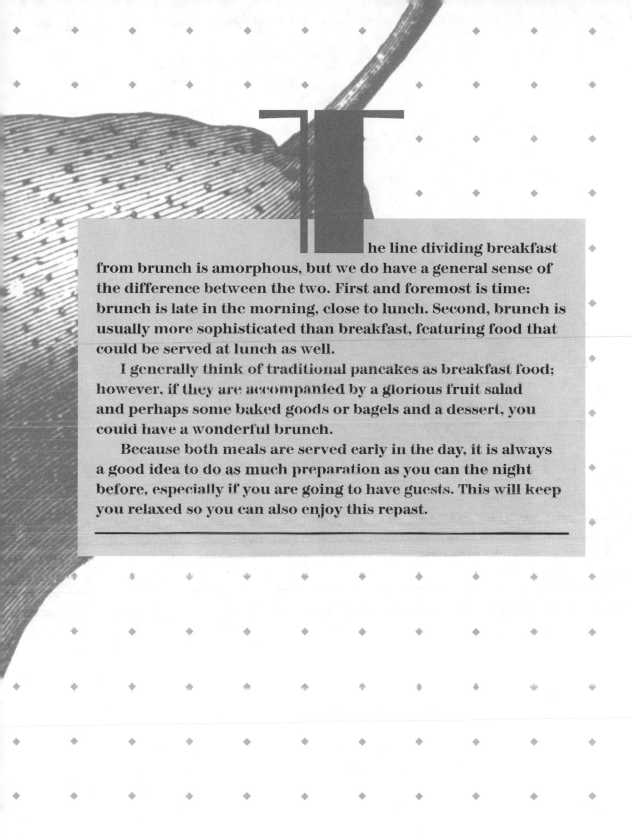

The line dividing breakfast from brunch is amorphous, but we do have a general sense of the difference between the two. First and foremost is time: brunch is late in the morning, close to lunch. Second, brunch is usually more sophisticated than breakfast, featuring food that could be served at lunch as well.

I generally think of traditional pancakes as breakfast food; however, if they are accompanied by a glorious fruit salad and perhaps some baked goods or bagels and a dessert, you could have a wonderful brunch.

Because both meals are served early in the day, it is always a good idea to do as much preparation as you can the night before, especially if you are going to have guests. This will keep you relaxed so you can also enjoy this repast.

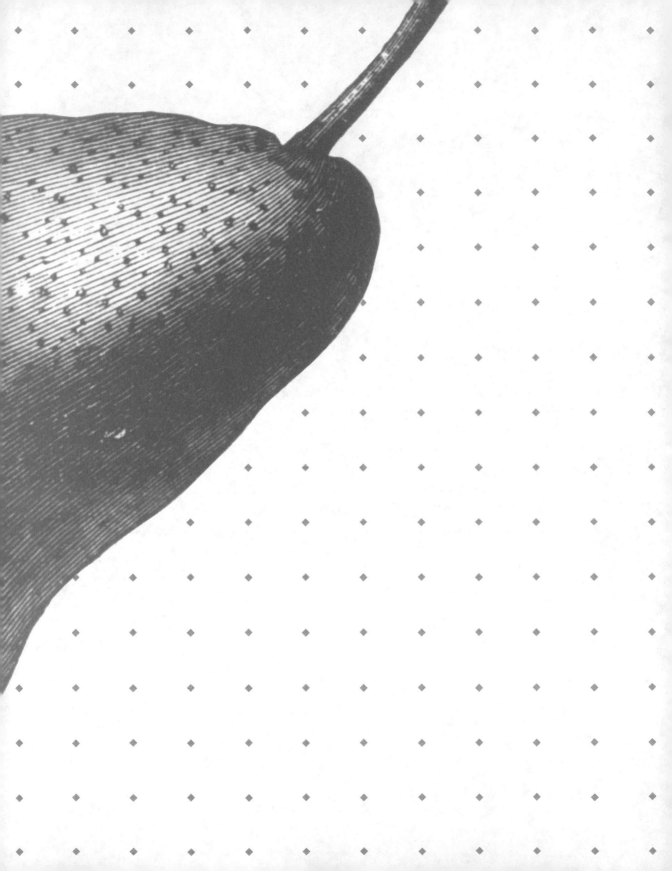

SOURDOUGH PANCAKES

These light, tasty sour-dough pancakes are quicker to prepare in the morning than traditional pancakes because half the work is done the day before.

THE STARTER

1 tablespoon active dry yeast

1½ cups warm water

2 teaspoons sugar

1 cup unbleached white flour

½ cup whole wheat flour

THE ADDITIONS

¾ teaspoon baking powder

¾ teaspoon salt

4 teaspoons sugar

2 eggs, lightly beaten

2 tablespoons milk

3 tablespoons butter, melted

Serves 4 to 0

1 Combine the yeast, water, and sugar in a large bowl and stir to blend. Let sit 5 minutes. Stir in the two flours and mix until smooth. Let sit, uncovered, for 2 hours. Cover the bowl with plastic wrap and refrigerate for 24 hours.

2 Whisk in the baking powder, salt, and sugar, then whisk in the eggs, milk, and butter; beat until smooth.

3 Heat a lightly greased skillet or griddle over medium heat. Add enough batter to make 4-inch pancakes and flip when bubbles have burst on the top of each pancake. They should be golden brown on each side when done. Serve with maple syrup.

OATMEAL PANCAKES WITH RASPBERRY HONEY

Adding oat flour to bread products gives them a wonderful flavor and texture, and these pancakes are a good example of that. In the past, only maple syrup would adorn my pancakes because I love its flavor so much, but this raspberry honey is so delicious and has such a captivating color that it has become a competing favorite.

RASPBERRY HONEY

1 cup fresh or frozen raspberries

1 cup honey

3 tablespoons water

½ teaspoon grated lemon rind

THE PANCAKES

½ cup oats

1 cup unbleached flour

½ teaspoon salt

3 tablespoons sugar

1¾ teaspoons baking powder

1 egg

3 tablespoons butter, melted and cooled

1½ cups low-fat milk

Serves 3 to 4

1 To make the raspberry honey, combine the berries, half the honey, and the water in a medium-size saucepan. Bring to a simmer and cook, stirring often, for 15 minutes.

2 Strain the honey through a sieve and press as many solids through as possible. Discard the seeds. Beat in the remaining honey and the lemon rind and let cool.

3 To make the pancakes, place the oats in a blender and grind until powdery. Pour them into a large bowl, then thoroughly mix in the flour, salt, sugar, and baking powder.

4 Beat the egg in a medium-size bowl. Beat in the butter and milk until blended. Pour this into the flour mixture and stir until thoroughly combined, but don't overmix it. Let the batter sit 5 minutes.

5 Heat a large skillet or griddle over medium heat until a drop of water sizzles when flicked on it. Make 3½-inch pancakes, flipping them over once bubbles have burst on the top. Serve with the raspberry honey.

APPLE PANCAKES

The memorable apple pancakes at Martin's restaurant in Great Barrington, Massachusetts, are the inspiration for these pancakes. They are always a big hit because the caramelized apples give them so much flavor. If you sauté the apples the night before, it will simplify your morning work. Also, don't hesitate to serve these for supper; they are the perfect comfort food.

THE APPLES

3 medium-size apples (any variety except Granny Smith or Golden Delicious, which are too firm)

1 tablespoon unsalted butter

1 tablespoon firmly packed brown sugar

½ teaspoon cinnamon

¼ teaspoon grated nutmeg

½ teaspoon vanilla extract

THE PANCAKES

1½ cups unbleached flour (or substitute ½ cup whole wheat flour for ½ cup white flour)

1½ teaspoons baking powder

1 tablespoon sugar

½ teaspoon salt

1 egg

1½ cups low-fat milk

3 tablespoons butter, melted and cooled

Serves 3 to 4

1 Peel and core the apples, then very thinly slice them.

2 Melt the butter in a large skillet over medium heat. Add the apple slices and sauté until they begin to soften, about 5 minutes. Add the brown sugar, cinnamon, and nutmeg and sauté, tossing often, until very tender, about 7 more minutes. Sprinkle on the vanilla, toss, then spoon onto a plate and let cool.

3 To make the batter, thoroughly combine the flour, baking powder, sugar, and salt in a large bowl. In a separate bowl, beat the egg, then stir in the milk and melted butter. Pour this into the flour mixture and stir until combined. Stir in the cooled apples.

4 Lightly oil a griddle or large skillet and heat over medium heat until it is hot enough for a drop of water to dance on it. Spoon on some batter to make 3-inch pancakes. Flip when bubbles form and burst on top. Cook until golden. Serve with maple syrup.

BAKED FRENCH TOAST

Quick

This has become one of my favorite breakfast preparations when entertaining because the little time needed to prepare this dish is spent the night before, thereby allowing me a hassle-free morning with a substantial breakfast. Great when you have houseguests.

Butter for greasing

6 slices firm bread (such as sourdough)

5 eggs

1½ cups low-fat milk

2 teaspoons vanilla extract

1 teaspoon ground cinnamon

⅛ teaspoon grated nutmeg

THE TOPPING

4 tablespoons unsalted butter, softened

⅓ cup firmly packed light brown sugar

½ cup finely chopped walnuts

Serves 4 to 6

1 Generously butter a $12 \times 7 \times 2$-inch baking dish (such as a rectangular Pyrex). Lay the bread slices in the dish, cutting slices to fill the spaces.

2 Beat the eggs in a large bowl. Beat in the milk, vanilla, cinnamon, and nutmeg. Pour over the bread, making sure it is submerged. Cover the dish and refrigerate overnight.

3 To make the topping, combine the butter, brown sugar, and walnuts in a small bowl. Keep at room temperature until you are ready to bake the French toast.

4 Preheat the oven to 350 degrees.

5 With a knife, spread the topping all over the bread. Bake 40 minutes, or until puffed and golden. Let sit 10 minutes before cutting. Cut into squares and serve with maple syrup. (Leftover French toast is delicious reheated; just bake until hot.)

CORN, RED PEPPER, AND SCALLION PANCAKES

Jam-packed with veg-
etables, these tasty pancakes need only a
spoonful of salsa and a dot of sour cream for
a special brunch or dinner offering. Great
served with home fries.

1 tablespoon vegetable oil

1 medium red bell pepper,
cored and finely diced

4 scallions, thinly sliced

4 eggs

⅔ cup milk

1¼ cups unbleached flour

1¼ teaspoons baking
powder

¾ teaspoon salt

1 teaspoon sugar

Freshly ground pepper

2 cups frozen corn kernels,
thawed

Vegetable oil for frying

Salsa

Sour cream

*Serves 3 to 4 (9 4-inch
pancakes)*

1 Heat the oil in a large skillet over medium heat.
Add the bell pepper and scallions and sauté
just until the pepper is tender, about 7 minutes.
Set aside to cool.

2 Beat the eggs in a large bowl. Beat in the milk.
Add the flour, baking powder, salt, sugar, and
pepper and mix just until combined. Stir in the
cooled vegetables and the corn.

3 Coat a large frying pan with a very thin layer
of oil and heat over medium heat until hot. Cook
about 3 pancakes at a time using about ¼ cup
batter per pancake. The pancakes are done when
they are golden brown on both sides and cooked
through. Serve with a large spoonful of salsa on
top of each pancake and a tiny spoonful of sour
cream on the salsa.

Note: Leftover uncooked batter can be refrigerated and used the next day.

MUSHROOM CROQUETTES

A *crisp coating encases a creamy center of mushrooms in a cheese sauce, making these croquettes a wonderful alternative to eggs for brunch. Make the filling the night before so you can have an easy morning before the guests arrive. For an accompaniment, toss diced sweet potatoes with oil and bake for 30 minutes.*

1 tablespoon olive oil

1 medium onion, very finely diced

1 pound mushrooms, finely chopped (4 cups)

½ teaspoon dried thyme

3 tablespoons unsalted butter

5 tablespoons unbleached flour

¾ cup low-fat milk

1 egg yolk

¼ cup grated Parmesan cheese

½ teaspoon salt

Freshly ground black pepper

Pinch of grated nutmeg

2 tablespoons minced fresh parsley

....

1 egg, beaten

1 cup bread crumbs

Oil for frying

Serves 4

1 Heat the oil in a large skillet over medium-high heat. Add the onion and sauté until tender, about 5 minutes. Stir in the mushrooms and thyme and cook, stirring often, until the mushrooms release their juices and then the juices evaporate, about 15 minutes. The mushrooms are done when they begin to stick to the pan. Remove the pan from the heat and let the mushrooms cool.

2 Melt the butter in a medium-size saucepan over medium heat. Whisk in the flour and cook, whisking constantly, for 2 minutes. Whisk in the milk and cook until it gets very thick, about 2 more minutes. Remove the sauce from the heat and let cool 5 minutes.

3 Whisk the egg yolk into the sauce. Using a spoon, stir in the Parmesan cheese, salt, pepper, nutmeg, and parsley. Stir in the mushrooms, then cover the pot and chill until very cold, at least 2 hours or up to 24 hours.

4 To bread the croquettes, place the beaten egg in a small soup bowl and place the bread crumbs in another small bowl. Using a ¼-cup measure, scoop up a scant ¼ cup of the mushroom mixture, roughly shape it into a 2½ × 3-inch log with your hands, then place it in the beaten egg. Roll it over to coat evenly, then roll it in the bread crumbs. Place the croquettes on a large plate as you finish breading them. These can be kept at room temperature for an hour before you fry them.

5 Pour about ¼ inch of oil into a large skillet. Heat over medium-high heat until the oil sizzles when a tiny bread crumb is dropped into it. In batches, fry the croquettes on both sides until golden brown. Drain on paper towels. You can keep the croquettes warm in a 325-degree oven up to 30 minutes.

VEGETABLE QUICHE WITH SMOKED CHEESE

Almost any combination of precooked vegetables would be delectable in this quiche. Strive for contrasting colors, and don't hesitate to try spinach, mushrooms, red pepper, or zucchini.

THE CRUST

Ice cubes

1 glass water

1 cup unbleached flour

¼ cup whole wheat flour

¼ teaspoon salt

5 tablespoons unsalted butter, chilled and cut into bits

2 tablespoons vegetable oil

THE FILLING

1 tablespoon olive oil

1 medium onion, finely diced

1 garlic clove, minced

½ cup diced yellow squash

1 cup tiny broccoli florets

1 tomato, seeded and diced

¼ teaspoon dried basil

¼ teaspoon dried marjoram

3 eggs

1¼ cups milk

½ teaspoon salt

1 To make the crust, place some ice cubes in a glass of water and set aside. In a large bowl, combine the two flours and salt. Add the butter bits and toss to coat. With your fingertips, quickly rub the butter into the flour until coarse crumbs form. You don't want the butter to be perfectly blended. Pour on the oil and toss to blend.

2 Sprinkle on 3 tablespoons of the ice water, toss, then gather the dough into a ball. If it is too dry, sprinkle on an additional tablespoon of water. Knead the dough two or three times to make it smooth. Gather it into a ball, flatten it into a disk, then wrap with plastic wrap. Chill 10 minutes, or until slightly firm.

3 On a lightly floured surface, roll the dough large enough to fit a 10-inch quiche pan. Fill the pan with the pastry, pushing it ¼ inch above the rim of the pan to allow for shrinkage. Prick all over with a fork. Freeze the crust for 30 minutes, or cover and freeze up to 1 month.

4 Preheat the oven to 375 degrees.

5 Line the piecrust with foil. Cover the bottom with pie weights or dried beans to prevent shrinkage. Bake the crust for 12 minutes, remove

Freshly ground pepper

**½ cup grated smoked
Gouda cheese**

½ cup grated Swiss cheese

Serves 4

the foil and weights, then bake 3 minutes more.
Let cool while making the filling.

6 Heat the oil in a large skillet over medium heat.
Add the onion and garlic and sauté for 5 minutes.
Stir in the squash, broccoli, and 2 tablespoons
of water. Cover the pan and steam until tender.
Remove the cover and boil away any remaining
water. Stir in the tomato and herbs and sauté
1 minute. Set aside to cool.

7 Beat the eggs in a large bowl. Beat in the milk,
salt, and pepper.

8 Sprinkle the smoked and Swiss cheeses over
the bottom of the piecrust. Arrange the vegetables
over the cheeses. Carefully pour in the egg mixture, being certain not to overfill the pie. (Leftover
custard can be baked in a buttered custard cup.)
Bake for 35 to 40 minutes, or until a knife
inserted in the center of the quiche comes out
clean and the top is golden. Let the quiche sit for
15 minutes before cutting and serving. Quiche
is most delicious served warm, not hot.

ZUCCHINI AND POTATO PANCAKES WITH TOMATO AND RED PEPPER SAUCE

You can grate the zucchini in advance, but don't make the batter until you are ready to start cooking. I like to serve egg noodles with these pancakes.

THE SAUCE

1 tablespoon olive oil

1 small onion, minced

1 small red bell pepper, cored and finely diced

1 large tomato, cored, seeded, and diced (1 cup)

Salt

Freshly ground pepper

THE PANCAKES

3 cups grated zucchini (2 medium)

1 8-ounce baking potato, peeled and grated

2 tablespoons grated onion

3 tablespoons unbleached flour

1 tablespoon grated Parmesan cheese

1 egg, beaten

½ teaspoon dried basil

½ teaspoon salt

Freshly ground pepper

Oil for frying

Serves 3 (12 3-inch pancakes)

1 To make the sauce, heat the oil in a medium skillet over medium heat. Add the onion and red pepper and sauté 5 minutes. Stir in the tomato and salt and pepper to taste and cook until there is a nice sauce consistency and the juices have thickened, about 15 minutes. Keep warm until needed.

2 To make the pancakes, place the zucchini in a cotton kitchen towel and gather it into a ball. Squeeze out all the juices. Place the zucchini in a large bowl.

3 Stir in all the remaining pancake ingredients except the oil. Heat a very thin layer of oil in a large skillet over medium-high heat. Fill a ¼-cup measure with batter for each pancake and drop on the skillet. Flatten with a spatula to make thin pancakes. Fry on both sides until a rich golden brown. As they finish cooking, keep warm on a baking sheet in a 350-degree oven until completed. Serve with a spoonful of sauce on each.

ESPECIALLY FOR ENTERTAINING

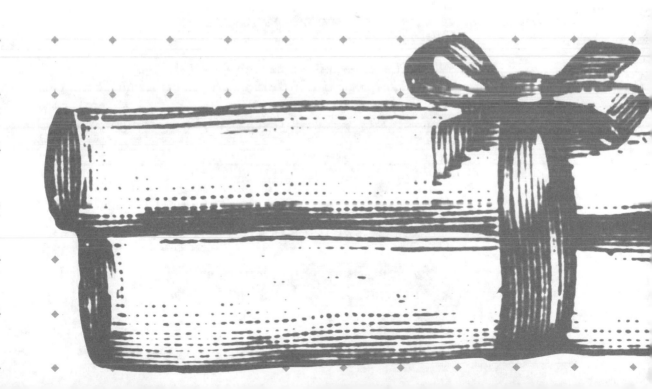

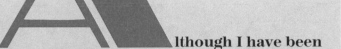

Although I have been exceedingly fond of quick recipes in recent years, every now and then I get the yen to prepare an elaborate meal for friends and immerse myself in the process of cooking. The recipes in this section are generally more involved than others in this book and are good choices when you want to serve something extra special.

When I taught cooking, I would always encourage my students to divide time-consuming recipes into segments. Rather than feel you have to cook uninterruptedly, start early in the day and perform a few steps like chopping vegetables and grating cheese, then come back to the recipe later. This approach makes demanding recipes quite easy.

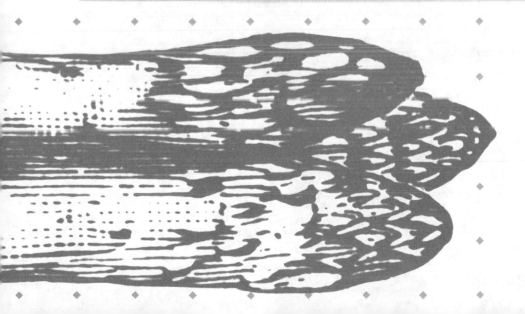

I have given suggestions for side dishes for most of these recipes. Add a salad and a special dessert and you'll have elegant meatless dinners.

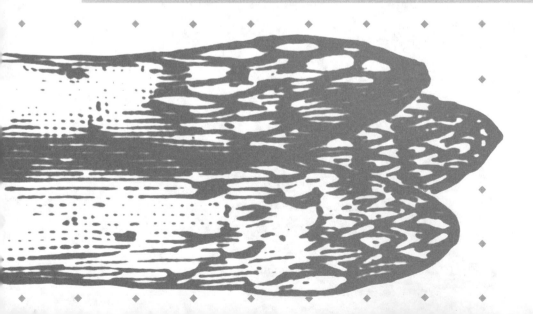

CARAMELIZED ONION TART

*Long slow cooking
gives the onions a rich brown color and a fabulous sweet flavor. Serve this tart alongside a
pilaf and perhaps a colorful steamed vegetable
such as green beans or carrots.*

3 tablespoons unsalted
butter

4 pounds onions, thinly
sliced (about 16 cups)

¼ teaspoon dried thyme

½ teaspoon salt

Freshly ground pepper

1 sheet frozen puff pastry
(half a 17¼-ounce box),
thawed

Serves 4 to 6

1 Melt the butter in a large pot over medium heat. Stir in the onions and thyme and cook, stirring frequently, until the onions are brown and jam-like, about 1 hour. Season with salt and pepper and scrape into a bowl to cool. (Can be prepared, cooled, covered, and chilled for up to 24 hours.)

2 Roll the puff pastry sheet into an 11-inch square. Place it in a 9-inch tart pan with a removable bottom and trim off the excess. Freeze 30 minutes, or place in a plastic bag and freeze up to 24 hours.

3 Preheat the oven to 425 degrees.

4 Scrape the onion mixture into the tart shell. Bake 25 minutes, or until the crust is golden brown. Cool slightly, then remove the outer rim. Serve warm rather than piping hot.

HOMEMADE MUSHROOM AND GOAT CHEESE RAVIOLI WITH GINGER CREAM SAUCE

The person who first thought of using wonton wrappers to make homemade ravioli and tortellini is brilliant. They are easy to use and make a delicate casing, thereby allowing you time to experiment with fillings. This is a wonderfully elegant dish—a good choice for a special occasion. Serve it with a salad of baby greens and some hot, crusty bread.

1 tablespoon olive oil

4 garlic cloves, minced

1 pound mushrooms, minced (about 4½ cups)

¼ teaspoon dried thyme

Pinch of grated nutmeg

⅛ teaspoon salt

Generous seasoning of freshly ground pepper

1 tablespoon minced fresh parsley

⅓ cup (packed) goat cheese

1 16-ounce package wonton wrappers (about 60 wrappers)

1 egg yolk, beaten with 1 teaspoon water (egg wash)

THE SAUCE

½ tablespoon unsalted butter

1 tablespoon minced fresh ginger

1 garlic clove, minced

1 To make the filling, heat the oil in a large skillet over medium-high heat. Add the garlic and cook until lightly golden, about 2 minutes. Do not let it brown. Stir in the mushrooms, thyme, nutmeg, salt, and pepper and sauté until the juices are released and then evaporate, about 15 minutes. The mixture will begin to stick to the pan when it is done.

2 Scrape the filling into a bowl and let it cool completely. Stir in the parsley and goat cheese.

3 Place the wonton wrappers and egg wash in front of you. Place one wrapper on a cutting board. Measure out 1 teaspoon of filling and put it on the center of the wrapper. Form it into a neat ball with your fingers. With a pastry brush, lightly brush some egg wash along the perimeter of the wrapper. Place another wrapper on top, then with your fingers seal the dough, keeping the ball intact while pressing out any air pockets.

4 With a 2½-inch round biscuit (pastry) cutter (or knife), cut out the ravioli and discard the scraps. Repeat with the remaining filling and wrappers.

½ tablespoon unbleached
flour

2 tablespoons pale dry
sherry, dry vermouth, or
dry white wine

⅔ cup whole milk

Salt

Freshly ground pepper

....

1 tablespoon minced fresh
parsley for garnish

Serves 4

You should have about 30 ravioli. As they are
completed, place them on a large platter, then
cover with plastic wrap. The ravioli can be
prepared up to 8 hours in advance and refrigerated. Bring to room temperature before cooking
because they should cook for 1 minute only
and cold ravioli requires longer cooking time.

5 To make the sauce, combine the butter, ginger,
and garlic in a small saucepan over medium
heat. Cook until the garlic begins to turn golden,
about 2 minutes. Whisk in the flour and cook
1 minute. Whisk in the sherry, milk, and salt
and pepper to taste and bring to a boil. Strain the
sauce into a small bowl and discard the ginger
and garlic.

6 To cook the ravioli, bring a large pot of water to
a boil. Drop in the ravioli, and after the water
returns to a boil, cook the ravioli just 1 minute.
Carefully pour the ravioli into a colander and let
drain.

7 Pour the sauce into the pot and heat just until it
begins to simmer. (If it is too thick, add a few
drops of milk.) Return the ravioli to the pot and
gently toss to coat. Serve garnished with the
parsley.

EGGPLANT ROLLATINI

This is a delicious dish. Its filling is somewhat firm compared to the traditional ricotta filling found in most eggplant rollatinis, and is far superior, I think. Because its preparation can be separated so easily into stages, it can be a hassle-free meal if you take advantage of these do-ahead tips. Up to 24 hours in advance, make the sauce, then cook the eggplant. Chill. Finally, make the filling and then assemble the rollatini. And don't hesitate to freeze the entire dish because it won't suffer a bit from it.

Steamed diced green beans or sautéed zucchini are lovely with this dish. You could also try buttered and parsleyed egg noodles for a more substantial addition.

THE SAUCE

2 tablespoons olive oil

3 garlic cloves, minced

1 28-ounce can crushed tomatoes

2 tablespoons red wine

1 teaspoon dried oregano

1 teaspoon dried basil

½ teaspoon salt

Liberal seasoning of freshly ground pepper

....

2 medium-size eggplants (about 2 pounds)

¾ cup bread crumbs

½ cup olive oil

THE FILLING

4 eggs

1 garlic clove, minced

1 To make the sauce, heat the olive oil in a medium-size saucepan over medium heat. Add the garlic and sauté just until it begins to turn golden. Do not let it get brown. Immediately stir in the tomatoes, wine, oregano, basil, salt, and pepper. Partially cover the pot to prevent the sauce from splattering all over the stove. Simmer, stirring occasionally, for 20 minutes. Set aside to cool.

2 To prepare the eggplants, cut off their ends. Cut them lengthwise into ¼-inch slices, keeping the skin on.

3 Preheat the broiler.

4 Pour the bread crumbs onto a large plate. With a pastry brush, coat both sides of each eggplant slice with a thin layer of olive oil, then dip the slices into the bread crumbs to coat them completely. In batches, place them on a cookie sheet and broil on both sides until golden brown

¾ cup finely chopped fresh parsley

¼ cup minced fresh basil, or 1 teaspoon dried

½ cup bread crumbs

¾ cup grated Parmesan cheese

1 cup grated part-skim mozzarella cheese

Serves 6

and very tender. Stack them on a platter after each batch is finished.

5 To make the filling, beat the eggs in a medium-size bowl. Beat in all the remaining filling ingredients except ½ cup of the mozzarella cheese.

6 Preheat the oven to 375 degrees.

7 Put a thin layer of the tomato sauce on the bottom of a $13 \times 9 \times 2$-inch baking dish. Divide the stuffing to match the number of eggplant slices. Place one portion of the stuffing at the end of an eggplant slice, then roll to cover. Place seam side down in the baking dish and proceed with the remaining eggplant slices.

8 Pour the remaining sauce over all the eggplant rolls, then sprinkle the remaining ½ cup of mozzarella on each roll. Cover the dish with foil.

9 Bake for 30 minutes, then remove the foil and bake an additional 10 minutes, or until hot and bubbly.

 Note: This dish may be prepared through step 8 up to 24 hours in advance and refrigerated, or frozen up to 2 weeks in advance. If frozen, let thaw in the refrigerator overnight before baking.

GRILLED POLENTA WITH ZUCCHINI AND SUN-DRIED TOMATOES

*A**dding a touch of heavy cream to this sauce makes it truly luscious and fit for a special occasion. If you don't have a grill, you can broil the polenta with equally good results.*

THE POLENTA

3½ cups vegetable stock

½ teaspoon salt

1 teaspoon finely chopped fresh rosemary, or ¼ teaspoon dried, crumbled

1 cup cornmeal

2 tablespoons unsalted butter

¼ cup grated Parmesan cheese

1 cup grated part-skim mozzarella cheese

2 tablespoons olive oil

THE SAUCE

½ cup sun-dried tomatoes (see note)

1 tablespoon olive oil

2 garlic cloves, minced

1 medium onion, finely diced

3 medium zucchini, cut in half lengthwise, then thinly sliced on the diagonal

⅓ cup heavy cream

1 To make the polenta, set aside a 10 × 10-inch shallow baking dish or other comparable dish. Bring the vegetable stock, salt, and rosemary to a boil in a medium-size saucepan. Reduce the heat to a simmer, then gradually sprinkle in the cornmeal, whisking constantly. Cook the polenta, whisking all the while, until it begins to pull away from the sides of the pan, about 7 minutes. Whisk in the butter, Parmesan cheese, and mozzarella cheese.

2 Scrape the polenta into the reserved baking dish and smooth over the top. Let cool for 10 minutes, then cover and chill for at least 1 hour, or up to 24 hours. When you are ready to begin cooking, cut the polenta into 8 squares. Lightly brush each side with the olive oil and place the squares on a baking sheet. Set aside while you make the sauce.

3 To make the sauce, place the sun-dried tomatoes in a bowl. Pour boiling water on them to cover. Let sit 10 minutes. Drain, then pat dry with paper towels. Slice the tomatoes into thin strips.

4 Heat the olive oil in a large skillet over medium-high heat. Add the garlic and onion and sauté

Salt

Liberal seasoning of freshly ground pepper

....

Fresh rosemary sprigs for garnish (optional)

Serves 4

for 5 minutes. Stir in the zucchini and sun-dried tomatoes and sauté until the zucchini is tender yet still slightly crunchy, about 7 minutes.

5 Meanwhile, grill or broil the polenta until golden brown on each side, about 10 minutes total. Place 2 squares of polenta on each serving plate.

6 Pour the cream into the zucchini mixture along with the salt and pepper. Let boil just until the sauce begins to thicken, about 1 minute. Spoon onto the polenta and garnish with fresh rosemary sprigs.

Note: If your sun-dried tomatoes are packed in oil, use only ⅓ cup. Omit cooking them in step 3; just slice them into strips.

SPINACH ENCHILADAS WITH ALMOND RED SAUCE

The addition of ground nuts to sauces is a Southwestern technique, which lends the sauce extra body and a richer flavor. I love these enchiladas and hope you will, too.

THE SAUCE

½ cup almonds

1 tablespoon olive oil

1 medium onion, minced

2 garlic cloves, minced

¼ teaspoon crushed red pepper flakes

2 cups tomato sauce (homemade or store-bought)

⅔ cup water

2 teaspoons paprika

THE FILLING

1 egg

1 15-ounce container part-skim ricotta cheese

1 10-ounce package frozen chopped spinach, thawed and pressed dry in a strainer

1 4-ounce can chopped green chilies, drained

2 tablespoons finely chopped cilantro

¼ teaspoon salt

Freshly ground pepper

1 Preheat the oven to 375 degrees.

2 To make the sauce, place the almonds in a shallow dish and toast until they are fragrant and begin to turn golden, about 5 minutes. Let cool, then grind until powdery in a blender. Set aside. Keep the oven on if you plan to cook the enchiladas right away.

3 Heat the oil in a medium-size saucepan over medium heat. Add the onion, garlic, and red pepper flakes and, stirring often, cook until the onion begins to brown, about 10 minutes. Stir in the tomato sauce, water, and paprika. Boil 2 minutes, then stir in the ground almonds. Remove from the heat.

4 To make the filling, beat the egg in a large bowl. Beat in all the remaining filling ingredients. Divide the filling into 8 portions.

5 Spoon a thin layer of sauce in a 9 × 13-inch baking dish. Place a tortilla on a plate, spoon a little sauce on it, and spread it around with the back of a spoon. Flip the tortilla over and repeat (this softens the tortilla and helps prevent it from breaking). Place an eighth of the spinach mixture along the edge of the tortilla, then roll it up to form a cylinder. Place in the baking dish, seam

8 6½-inch flour tortillas

1 cup grated Monterey Jack cheese

Serves 4

side down, and repeat with the remaining tortillas and filling.

6 Pour the remaining sauce over the enchiladas, then sprinkle on the grated cheese. Cover the dish with foil.

7 Bake for 30 minutes, or until bubbly.

Note: May be prepared up to 8 hours in advance through step 6. Bring to room temperature before baking.

STUFFED BASIL CRÊPES WITH ROASTED RED PEPPER SAUCE

Stuffed with a zucchini and goat cheese filling, these crêpes can be prepared in stages, making this elegant dish seem easy. Couscous is a good side dish.

THE CREPES

1 egg

½ cup unbleached flour

¼ teaspoon salt

½ cup plus 2 tablespoons milk

2 tablespoons butter, melted

1½ tablespoons minced fresh basil, or 1 teaspoon dried

Butter or oil for greasing pan

THE FILLING

1 tablespoon olive oil

2 garlic cloves, minced

1 medium onion, finely diced

1 tomato, cored, seeded, and finely diced

¼ teaspoon fennel seed, crushed

2 medium zucchini, cut lengthwise into sixths and thinly sliced (4 cups)

Salt

Generous seasoning of freshly ground pepper

1 To make the crêpes, combine the egg, flour, salt, milk, and melted butter in a blender and blend until smooth. Pour the batter into a bowl and stir in the basil.

2 Heat an 8-inch omelet pan or nonstick skillet over medium-high heat and lightly grease the pan. With a measuring spoon, pour a scant 2 tablespoons of batter into the pan and swirl it around to coat the entire surface. Cook the crêpe for about 2 minutes, or until lightly browned. Flip and cook about 1 more minute. Place the cooked crêpe on a sheet of wax paper and repeat until all the batter has been used. You should have 8 crêpes. They can be stacked on each other to cool. (The crêpes may be prepared up to 48 hours in advance, wrapped, and refrigerated.)

3 To make the filling, heat the olive oil in a large skillet over medium-high heat. Add the garlic and onion and sauté for 5 minutes, or until the onion begins to get tender. Stir in the tomato and fennel and cook 1 minute. Stir in the zucchini and cook, stirring often, until tender, about 10 minutes. Season with salt and pepper to taste. (The filling may be made up to 48 hours in advance and chilled.)

THE SAUCE

1 7-ounce jar roasted red peppers, well drained and patted dry (1 cup)

¼ cup tomato sauce (homemade or store-bought)

1 garlic clove, minced

Dash of cayenne

Salt

....

6 ounces goat cheese, crumbled (about 1 cup)

Serves 4

4 To make the sauce, combine the peppers, tomato sauce, garlic, cayenne, and salt in a blender and purée. Pour into a small saucepan to heat at serving time.

5 Preheat the oven to 300 degrees.

6 To assemble the crêpes, lightly butter a 12 × 7 × 2-inch baking dish or one of similar size. One side of each crêpe will be more attractive and herb-flecked. Place this side down on a surface so it is on the outside. Spoon an eighth of the zucchini mixture along the center of the crêpe. Place some goat cheese on top of the filling, then roll the crêpe to make a log. Place seam side down in the baking dish. Repeat with all the crêpes.

7 Lay a lightly buttered sheet of wax paper on the crêpes. Cover the dish with aluminum foil. Bake 20 to 30 minutes, or until hot throughout.

8 Meanwhile, gently heat the sauce just until hot. Serve 2 crêpes on each plate with some sauce spooned on.

POLENTA TIMBALES WITH SPICY MUSHROOM SAUCE

These timbales are an ideal dish for entertaining because they are at once beautiful and delicate and also very satisfying. The bonus is that almost all the steps can be prepared in advance.

THE POLENTA

2 cups low-fat milk

2 cups water

1¼ cups cornmeal

¼ cup sour cream

¼ cup grated Parmesan cheese

½ teaspoon salt

⅛ teaspoon grated nutmeg

Freshly ground pepper

1 cup (4 ounces) finely diced Italian fontina cheese, plus 8 thin 1-inch-square slices Italian fontina cheese

THE SAUCE

2 tablespoons olive oil

1 medium onion, minced

4 garlic cloves, minced

¼ teaspoon crushed red pepper flakes

1 pound mushrooms, quartered or cut into eighths (about 7 cups)

1 28-ounce can imported plum tomatoes, finely chopped with their juice

1 Place 8 custard cups or ramekins in a handy spot to pour the polenta into when it's cooked. Arrange all the polenta ingredients in front of you before you begin cooking. Bring the milk and water to a boil in a medium-size heavy-bottomed saucepan. Reduce the heat to low, then slowly drizzle in the cornmeal, beating all the while with a wire whisk. Whisk constantly until the polenta tears away from the sides of the pot, about 5 minutes.

2 Remove from the heat and whisk in the sour cream, Parmesan cheese, salt, nutmeg, and pepper. Stir in the cubed fontina just until the cubes are evenly distributed (they shouldn't melt much). Quickly spoon the mixture into the custard cups, then smooth over the tops of the timbales with the back of a spoon, or overfill them and scrape off the excess with a knife. Let the timbales sit for 15 minutes. (The timbales may be prepared in advance up to this point, covered, and refrigerated for up to 24 hours.)

3 To make the sauce, heat the olive oil over medium-high heat in a large skillet. Add the onion, garlic, and red pepper flakes and cook, stirring often, until the onion is tender, about 7 minutes. Add the mushrooms and sauté until

1 tablespoon tomato paste

½ teaspoon salt

Liberal seasoning of
freshly ground pepper

1½ tablespoons minced
fresh parsley

Serves 4

the juices are released and then evaporated, about 15 minutes.

4 Stir in the tomatoes, tomato paste, salt, and pepper. Cook, stirring occasionally, until the sauce is thick, about 25 minutes. (The sauce may be prepared up to 24 hours in advance and refrigerated.)

5 Preheat the oven to 400 degrees. Generously butter a shallow broilerproof baking dish that's large enough to hold the 8 timbales.

6 Run a knife around each timbale to loosen it from the custard cup, then invert into the baking dish. Place a slice of the remaining cheese on top of each timbale. Bake for 15 minutes, then place under the broiler for 3 minutes, or until the cheese is bubbly. Remove from the oven and spread the cheese more evenly over the timbales. Broil 2 minutes more, or until golden.

7 If the sauce has become too thick again, thin it with a few more tablespoons of water. Stir in the minced parsley. Serve 2 timbales per person with the mushroom sauce surrounding them.

SPINACH AND GORGONZOLA RISOTTO

The characteristic creaminess of a risotto is achieved by ladling small amounts of stock into rice and stirring until it is absorbed before adding more stock. It is not difficult to do, but it is a last-minute dish that requires your full attention for about 40 minutes. You can chat with guests while performing this task, or pull up a stool and read a good book while stirring with your book-free hand. A special salad made with baby greens is all you need to accompany this luscious dish, but plan to serve it after the risotto.

4½ cups vegetable stock

⅛ teaspoon grated nutmeg

½ teaspoon salt

Freshly ground pepper

1 tablespoon unsalted butter

1 medium onion, minced

2 garlic cloves, minced

1 cup (3 ounces) thinly sliced mushrooms

1 cup arborio rice (see note)

3 cups (3 ounces) lightly packed spinach leaves, torn into small pieces

2 tablespoons golden raisins

2 ounces (about ½ cup) crumbled Gorgonzola cheese, or other blue cheese

½ cup grated Parmesan cheese

1 Combine the stock, nutmeg, salt, and pepper in a medium-size saucepan and heat just until hot. Reduce the heat to low and keep hot while you make the risotto.

2 In another medium-size, heavy-bottomed saucepan, melt the butter over medium-high heat. Add the onion and garlic and sauté, tossing often, until the onion begins to brown, about 7 minutes.

3 Stir in the mushrooms and cook until the mushrooms are brown and their juices have been released and then evaporated, about 10 minutes. Stir often. Stir in the rice and cook 2 minutes, stirring constantly to coat the grains evenly and cause them to become almost translucent.

4 Reduce the heat to medium. Fill a ½-cup ladle with hot stock and pour it on the rice mixture. Stir constantly until the liquid is absorbed, about 4 minutes. Add another ½ cup of stock and stir until it is absorbed. Keep repeating this procedure, making sure not to add stock until the

Serves 3 (can easily be doubled)

previous ladleful of stock has been absorbed. Each ladleful should take about 4 minutes.

5 When about two-thirds of the stock has been used, stir in the spinach and raisins. Continue to add the stock as described above. When 1 ladleful of stock remains, taste the rice. The grains should be tender but still slightly chewy—that is, al dente. If they are hard, add a ½ cup of warm water and test again after it has been absorbed. Before the last ladleful of stock has been added, stir in the Gorgonzola, Parmesan cheese, and last bit of stock. Stir 1 to 2 minutes, or until thick and creamy. Serve immediately.

Note: Arborio is an imported Italian rice with short, fat grains and a lot of starch. It's available at specialty food shops and many natural foods stores.

RISOTTO PRIMAVERA

Asparagus and peas lend a spring accent to this colorful risotto, but actually it can be made during any season now that asparagus is practically a year-round vegetable.

4½ cups vegetable stock

½ teaspoon salt

Generous seasoning of freshly ground pepper

2 tablespoons olive oil

1 carrot, very thinly sliced

5 asparagus stalks, peeled and cut into 1-inch pieces

1 red bell pepper, cut into ½-inch dice

½ cup fresh peas or thawed frozen peas

1 medium onion, minced

2 garlic cloves, minced

1 cup arborio rice (see note, page 191)

1 tablespoon finely shredded fresh basil, or ½ teaspoon dried

½ cup grated Parmesan cheese

Serves 3

1 Combine the stock, salt, and pepper in a medium-size saucepan (on a back burner) and bring to a simmer. Reduce the heat to low and keep hot while making the risotto.

2 Heat 1 tablespoon of the oil in a medium-size skillet over medium heat. Add the sliced carrot and sauté 1 minute. Stir in the asparagus and sauté 2 more minutes. Add the red pepper and fresh peas (if you are using them) and cook about 3 more minutes, or until the vegetables are tender but not mushy. If you are using frozen peas, add them now, then remove the pan from the heat. They do not need to cook.

3 In a heavy-bottomed medium-size saucepan, heat the remaining tablespoon of olive oil over medium heat. Add the onion and garlic and cook, stirring often, until the onion begins to brown, about 7 minutes. Stir in the rice and sauté 2 minutes, stirring constantly.

4 Fill a ½-cup ladle with stock and pour it on the rice. Stir constantly until the liquid is absorbed, about 4 minutes. Add another ½ cup of stock and stir until it is absorbed. Keep repeating this procedure, making sure not to add stock until the previous ladleful has been absorbed. It should take about 4 minutes for each ladleful of stock. Regulate the heat accordingly.

5 When one ladleful of stock remains, taste the rice. The grains should be tender but still slightly chewy. If they are hard, add ½ cup of warm water and test again after it has been absorbed. Before adding the last ladleful of stock, stir in the vegetables, basil, and Parmesan cheese, then the remaining stock. Stir 1 to 2 minutes, or until thick and creamy. Serve immediately.

BAKED STUFFED RED PEPPERS

*S*pinach fettuccine and smoked cheese are the main components of this highly flavorful stuffing, making these brilliant red peppers a feast for the eyes as well as the appetite. Because they are so substantial, all you need is some steamed summer squash to sit alongside them.

4 large red bell peppers

¼ pound spinach fettuccine

1 cup part-skim ricotta cheese

¼ cup plus 2 tablespoons low-fat milk

1 cup grated smoked cheese (such as smoked Gouda)

1 cup grated part-skim mozzarella cheese

2 scallions, very thinly sliced

½ teaspoon salt

Generous seasoning of freshly ground pepper

Olive oil for greasing

Serves 4

1 Slice the tops off the peppers (save these scraps for another use). Pull out the seeds and fibrous insides of each pepper and discard. To make each pepper sit steadily upright, slice a very thin piece off each bottom.

2 Bring a large pot of water to a boil. Drop the peppers in and let the water return to a boil. Cook 5 minutes, then remove the peppers with tongs. Invert them on a kitchen towel and let them drain and cool.

3 Return the water to a rapid boil. Cook the fettuccine for 7 minutes, or until al dente. Drain in a colander. You need about 2 cups fettuccine.

4 To make the stuffing, beat the ricotta with the milk in a large bowl. Stir in both cheeses, the scallions, salt, and pepper. Cut the fettuccine a few times with two knives to shorten the strands. Stir the fettuccine into the cheese mixture.

5 Preheat the oven to 375 degrees.

6 Rub a little olive oil all over the outside of each pepper. Stuff each pepper with the fettuccine mixture. Smooth over the tops by pressing down the stuffing. Place the peppers in a lightly oiled, shallow baking dish, such as a $12 \times 7 \times 2$-inch

Pyrex dish. Bake for 30 minutes, or until hot, bubbly, and lightly browned.

〰 ***Note:*** May be prepared, covered, and refrigerated up to 24 hours in advance. Bring to room temperature before cooking.

STUFFED YELLOW PEPPERS WITH TOMATO-BASIL SALSA

I like to make this tasty dish at the height of summer when the cost of yellow peppers is reasonable and tomatoes and basil are at their prime. The white bean and zucchini stuffing makes them substantial, so all you need for accompaniments are a salad and some crusty bread.

4 large yellow bell peppers

1 tablespoon olive oil, plus extra for greasing

3 garlic cloves, minced

2 medium zucchini, cut lengthwise into sixths and thinly sliced (2 cups sliced)

1 15-ounce can cannellini (white kidney beans)

¼ teaspoon powdered sage

⅓ cup grated Parmesan cheese

⅔ cup grated fontina, Monterey Jack, or Muenster cheese

Salt

Generous seasoning of freshly ground black pepper

THE SALSA

1 large ripe tomato, very finely diced (1 cup)

1 garlic clove, minced

½ cup finely shredded fresh basil

1 Cut the tops off the peppers. Cut any flesh away from the stem, finely dice it, and set aside. Discard the stem. Pull out the seeds and fibrous interior of the peppers and discard them.

2 Bring a large pot of water to a boil. Drop in the pepper shells and let the water return to a boil. Cook the peppers for 5 minutes. Remove them with tongs and let drain upside down.

3 Preheat the oven to 375 degrees.

4 Heat the tablespoon of oil in a large skillet over medium heat. Add the garlic and cook 1 minute. Stir in the zucchini and diced peppers and cook until tender yet still slightly crunchy. Remove from the heat, then stir in the cannellini, sage, two cheeses, salt, and pepper.

5 Lightly oil a shallow baking dish large enough to hold the peppers. Divide the vegetable-bean mixture into four, then stuff each pepper with it. Place in the baking dish. (May be prepared to this point and chilled up to 24 hours in advance.) Bake 30 minutes, or until piping hot and beginning to brown.

8 oil-cured black olives, pitted and chopped (see note, page 25)

2 teaspoons olive oil

2 teaspoons balsamic vinegar

Salt

Freshly ground black pepper

Serves 4

6 Meanwhile, combine all the salsa ingredients in a bowl. Let sit at room temperature until ready to use. Pass the salsa at the table to spoon onto the peppers.

EGGPLANT TART IN PUFF PASTRY

The deep meaty flavor
and garlicky overtones of this eggplant filling
are a nice match for delicate puff pastry. Pasta
would make a great side dish; try angel hair
with minced parsley or orzo with bits of sautéed
tomato mixed in.

1 sheet frozen puff pastry
(half a 17¼-ounce box),
thawed

....

2 tablespoons olive oil

1 medium onion, very
finely diced

4 garlic cloves, minced

1 16-ounce can tomatoes,
finely chopped and well
drained

1 large (1½ pounds)
eggplant, peeled and cut
into ¼-inch dice

1 green pepper, cut into
¼-inch dice

¼ cup finely chopped fresh
basil, or 1½ teaspoons
dried

¾ teaspoon salt

Generous seasoning of
freshly ground pepper

2 eggs

¼ cup grated Parmesan
cheese

1 Roll the puff pastry into an 11-inch square.
Place it in a 9-inch tart pan with a removable bottom and trim off the excess. Cover and freeze
for 30 minutes, or place in a plastic bag and freeze
up to 24 hours.

2 To make the filling, heat the olive oil in a large
skillet over medium heat. Add the onion and
garlic and cook 5 minutes, tossing often. Add the
tomatoes and sauté 5 more minutes.

3 Stir in the eggplant, green pepper, basil, salt,
and pepper and toss well. Cover the pan and cook
about 20 minutes, or until the eggplant is tender.
Remove from the heat and cool slightly.

4 Place two-thirds of the eggplant mixture, the
eggs, and the Parmesan cheese in a food processor
or blender and purée. Scrape the mixture back
into the skillet and mix with the reserved
eggplant.

5 Preheat the oven to 425 degrees.

6 Spoon the eggplant mixture into the frozen tart
shell and smooth over the top. In a small bowl,
combine the bread crumbs, Parmesan cheese,
garlic, parsley, and melted butter. Sprinkle evenly
over the tart.

CRUMB TOPPING (PERSILLADE)

1 tablespoon bread crumbs

1 tablespoon grated Parmesan cheese

1 garlic clove, minced

2 tablespoons minced fresh parsley

1 tablespoon unsalted butter, melted

Serves 4 to 6

7 Bake 25 minutes, or until a rich golden brown. Remove the outer rim of the tart pan and let the tart sit for 10 minutes before cutting into wedges.

SPINACH LOAF WITH CURRIED CREAM SAUCE

Buttered egg noodles
go very well with this savory loaf. Try sautéing
bits of red pepper or tomato and adding
them to noodles before serving; this will lend
an attractive splash of color.

2 pounds loose fresh
spinach, or 2 10-ounce
packages fresh spinach, or
2 10-ounce packages frozen
chopped spinach, thawed

1 tablespoon unsalted
butter

1 medium onion, minced

1 carrot, grated

3 eggs, beaten

1 cup low-fat milk

½ cup bread crumbs

3 tablespoons grated
Parmesan cheese

¼ teaspoon grated nutmeg

½ teaspoon salt

Freshly ground pepper

THE SAUCE

1½ tablespoons unsalted
butter

1 teaspoon curry powder

2 tablespoons unbleached
flour

2 cups milk

Dash of cayenne

Salt

Serves 4 to 6

1 If you are using fresh spinach, discard the stems, wash the leaves thoroughly, and drain them. Place the spinach in a large covered skillet or pot with only the water that clings to them. Cook until the spinach just wilts. Let cool; squeeze out the moisture with your hands. Finely chop the spinach. If you are using frozen spinach, just squeeze out all the moisture between your hands. Put it in a large bowl.

2 Heat the butter in a small skillet. Sauté the onion until tender. Combine with the spinach. Stir in the carrot, eggs, milk, bread crumbs, cheese, nutmeg, salt, and pepper to taste.

3 Preheat the oven to 375 degrees. Generously butter a 9 × 5-inch loaf pan. Line it with wax paper, then butter the paper.

4 Spoon the spinach mixture into the pan and smooth the top. Cover loosely with foil. Place the dish in a larger baking dish and fill with 1 inch of hot water.

5 Bake for 1½ hours, or until a knife inserted in the center of the loaf comes out clean. If a lot of water evaporates before the cooking time is up, add more hot water to keep it at a depth of 1 inch. Let sit for 10 minutes before unmolding onto a platter.

6 To make the sauce, melt the butter in a medium-size saucepan over medium heat. Whisk in the curry powder and flour and cook for 2 minutes, whisking constantly. Whisk in the milk, cayenne, and salt. Cook, whisking often, until the sauce comes to a boil.

7 Slice the loaf and serve with sauce spooned on each slice.

EGGPLANT STEAKS WITH PEPPERS AND TANGY BASIL SAUCE

Here's an attractive and delicious dish that can be prepared in easy stages and reheated. Rounds of crumb-coated broiled eggplant are topped with a colorful pepper sauté, then drizzled with a spoonful of garlicky basil sauce. Serve with a lightly buttered starch such as egg noodles, rice, or couscous.

THE PEPPERS

1 tablespoon olive oil

4 garlic cloves, minced

1 medium onion, halved and thinly sliced

1 green bell pepper, cored, halved, and thinly sliced

1 red bell pepper, cored, halved, and thinly sliced

2 tomatoes, cored, seeded, and finely diced

2 teaspoons drained capers

Salt

Generous seasoning of freshly ground pepper

THE SAUCE

1 cup low-fat yogurt

1 garlic clove, pressed or minced

¼ cup finely chopped fresh basil

Salt

Freshly ground pepper

1 To make the pepper sauté, heat the olive oil in a large skillet over medium-high heat. Add the garlic and onion and sauté, tossing often, for 10 minutes, or until the onion is tender.

2 Mix in the peppers, tomatoes, capers, salt, and pepper and cook about 20 minutes, or until the peppers are very tender and the mixture is jamlike. Stir often so that everything cooks evenly. The peppers can be cooked up to 8 hours in advance and reheated. Add a few drops of water if the mixture sticks to the pan.

3 Meanwhile, make the basil sauce by combining all the sauce ingredients in a small bowl. If made well in advance, keep chilled; otherwise, keep at room temperature to serve cool, not cold.

4 To cook the eggplant, preheat the broiler. With a pastry brush, lightly coat both sides of each eggplant slice with some olive oil, then coat the slices with the bread crumbs. Place on a baking sheet. Broil until golden brown on both sides, turning over as necessary. The eggplant can be prepared up to 24 hours in advance and reheated before serving.

THE EGGPLANT

1 medium (1¼ pounds) eggplant, skin left on and sliced ¾ inch thick

3 tablespoons olive oil

⅓ cup bread crumbs

Serves 4

5 To serve, place a few eggpl serving plate. Top with some then drizzle with a spoonful of

1 tab
butt

2 m
cho

1 p
fin

1
(1

2

USHROOM CUTLETS WITH SPICY CREAM SAUCE

These tasty pancakes remind me of sausage patties because of their texture and spicy overtones. You can serve them with a vegetable or noodle side dish, or alongside scrambled eggs for a breakfast treat. In either case, don't omit the sauce; it is simple yet hauntingly good.

...lespoon unsalted
...er

...dium onions, finely
...pped

...ound mushrooms,
...ely chopped

...up diced cooked potato
...medium)

...eggs

1¼ cup bread crumbs

2 tablespoons minced fresh parsley

1 cup grated Swiss cheese

½ teaspoon dried thyme

⅛ teaspoon celery seed

¾ teaspoon salt

Liberal seasoning of freshly ground pepper

Dash of cayenne

Oil for greasing

THE SAUCE

½ cup sour cream

½ cup medium-hot salsa

Serves 4 (11 to 12 cutlets)

1 Heat the butter in a large skillet over medium heat. Add the onions and sauté until tender, about 10 minutes. Raise the heat to medium-high and stir in the mushrooms. Cook, stirring often, until the juices have evaporated and the mixture begins to stick to the pan, 10 to 15 minutes.

2 Place in a food processor along with the potato and eggs and process until smooth. Scrape into a large bowl and let cool to room temperature. Stir in the remaining pancake ingredients except the oil.

3 Preheat the oven to 350 degrees. Generously oil a baking sheet.

4 Scoop the mixture into a ⅓-cup measure and scrape off the excess. Drop onto the baking sheet and flatten slightly. (You might have to use two baking sheets or cook these in two batches.) Bake 15 minutes, flip, then bake 15 additional minutes. They should be golden brown when done.

5 To make the sauce, beat together the sour cream and salsa. Serve a spoonful of sauce on each cutlet.

Note: May be prepared through step 2 up to 24 hours in advance. Keep covered and refrigerated.

INDEX